A Pea In My Pod:

The natural approach to pregnancy and motherhood

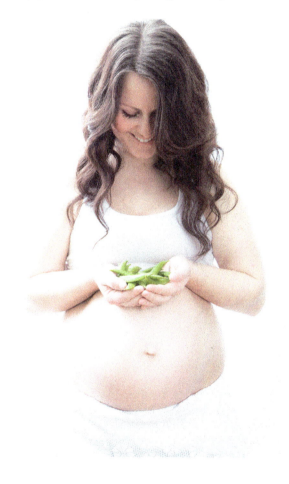

A holistic nutrition and lifestyle guide on fertility, pregnancy, birth, post-partum and childhood

BY THERESA MARTINS, R.H.N.

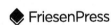

Suite 300 - 990 Fort St
Victoria, BC, Canada, V8V 3K2
www.friesenpress.com

Copyright © 2015 by Theresa Martins, R.H.N.
First Edition — 2015

All rights reserved.

No part of this publication may be reproduced in any form, or by any means, electronic or mechanical, including photocopying, recording, or any information browsing, storage, or retrieval system, without permission in writing from FriesenPress.

ISBN
978-1-4602-6949-7 (Hardcover)
978-1-4602-6950-3 (Paperback)
978-1-4602-6951-0 (eBook)

1. Health & Fitness, Pregnancy & Childbirth

Distributed to the trade by The Ingram Book Company

Table of Contents

A Little Intro!   ix

Chapter 1 - Preconception:
The Easy and the Hard Way   1

    Preparing the mind and body   2

    Power of digestion   3

    Food for thought   4

    What is really in your food?   5

    The "free" word   6

    The sugar effect   6

    Sugar by any other name   9

    The dirty dozen   13

    A gentle detox   14

    Ride the whole foods wave   17

Chapter 2 - "F" Is for Fertility   19

    Fertility food and what to watch out for   19

    Healthy and not-so-healthy packaged foods   20

    The lowdown on food additives   20

    Supplementations   22

    Synthetic vs. Natural   23

       The magic pill   23

       "C" is for conception   23

       The miraculous plant   24

    Exercise and alternative medicine   24

    Traditional Chinese medicine 25

    Visit the chiropractor 25

    See a nutritionist 25

Chapter 3 - What You Need to Know in Your First Trimester 27

    Honey, I'm pregnant! 27

    Midwife or doctor? 28

    The reality 29

    Morning sickness: Am I supposed to feel like this? 30

    The essentials 32

    Prevention of miscarriages 34

    Necessary avoidances 35

    Necessary Additives 36

Chapter 4 - What You Need to Know in Your Second Trimester 37

    Upping the calories 38

    The truth about gestational diabetes 39

        Who is at risk for developing GD? 39

        Prevention and management 39

        What can I expect if I develop GD? 40

        Foods to avoid 40

Chapter 5 - What You Need to Know in Your Third Trimester 41

    Pesky symptoms 42

    Pumping the iron 43

        Developing anemia 43

        Symptoms 43

Risks *44*

Foods to include *44*

Chapter 6 - No Meat Mommies — 45

Balance and food pairing — 45

It's all about the fat — 47

Fat deficiencies — *47*

Fat-soluble vitamins — *48*

Vitamins and minerals — 48

Chapter 7 - Mind and Body Detox — 51

Environmental toxins — 51

What to avoid — *51*

What's wrong with these toxins? — *52*

D.I.Y.M: Do it yourself mamas! — 53

All-purpose cleaning spray — 53

Mirror cleaner — 54

Organic homemade lotion — 54

"No poo" shampoo — 54

Epsom salt bath soak — 55

Organic baby oil — 55

Baby bum powder — 55

Herbal healing baby wipes — 55

Stress mess — 56

Coping mechanisms — 56

Chapter 8 - 35 Weeks and Up — 59

Birth prep — 60

Bring the bag — 61

Natural induction — 62

Birthing techniques	65
Push it, push it real good!	69

Chapter 9 - Welcome Baby — 71

Breastfeeding	71
Is breast the best?	71
Benefits of breastfeeding	73
Essentials in breast milk	74
Essentials in breast milk	75
What to include in your diet while nursing	76
What to avoid while nursing	76
Colic	77
What is colic?	78
Causes	78
Coping	79

Chapter 10 - Boobs and Barbells — 81

Nursing and exercise	81
Food first	81
Holistic Food Guide	84
Exercise	86

Chapter 11 - Moving On Up From Milk — 88

When to begin	89
Feeding time and first foods	90
Feeding plan for baby	91
Best solid foods from age 6 months to 1 year	91
The Moo	92
Soy	93
Dairy alternatives	94

Hydration	94
Infant supplements	95
Constipation	96
Symptoms	*96*
Causes	*96*
How to treat constipation	*97*

Chapter 12 - Food Allergies — 99

Hidden food allergies!	99
Allergy elimination diet	100

Chapter 13 - My Not-so-little Baby: Nutrition for the Growing Toddler and Child — 102

Quality over quantity	102
Up it to gain it	103
Let's get fat: The benefits of essential fatty acids (EFA'S)	104
The RDA	104
Fussy eaters	106

Chapter 14 - Veggie Baby — 108

No meat, no problem	108
What is vegetarian?	109
What is a vegan?	109
Getting enough: Balance is key	110
Hydration for your growing child	111

Chapter 15 - Eating for Mental Health — 113

What is autism?	113
What is ADHD?	114

The GFCF diet	114

Chapter 16 - Recipes and Meal Plan — **116**

7-Day sample meal plan	117
Family recipes	121
Smoothies and Juices and Bevies	*121*
Breakfast	*125*
Main Dishes	*127*
Side dishes	*130*
Salads	*132*
Soups and stews	*135*
Desserts	*139*
Condiments and dressing	*143*
Snacks	*148*
Baby food Recipes	152
Babies 6-8 months old	*152*
Babies 8-11 months old	*154*
Toddler Recipes (12 months and up)	156

Chapter 17 - FITNESS 101:
Prenatal and Postnatal Workouts — **161**

About the trainer	161
Prenatal exercises	162
Post-natal exercises	170

Image Credits — **185**

A Little Intro!

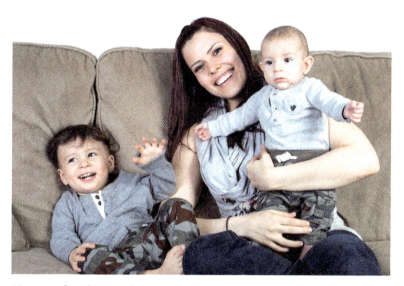

You come first photography

Many future mamas, mamas to be, and mamas already, may not be aware of the importance of nutrition for themselves, their unborn babies, and their young children. Even after years of working as a Registered Holistic Nutritionist and helping many of my clients learn about health and wellness before, during, and after pregnancy, I felt it still wasn't enough for me. I wanted the voice of holistic health to be heard by caring mothers and mothers-to-be everywhere.

Nutrition plays one of the most vital roles in fertility, pregnancy, and postpartum care. Our body is the temple in which our baby is kept sacred for 9 months. Therefore, we need to be the God of our temple and give it all we have to keep it strong, beautiful, and safe.

Throughout my book, I cover many important topics including: pre-pregnancy and the nutrients that you must feed your body in order to have an easy, successful conception; how to boost fertility if you are struggling with becoming pregnant; and how to eat properly when your baby is growing, gaining strength, and preparing for the journey outside the womb.

I also explore further into post pregnancy and how to heal and re-nourish your body after birth, gain back your confidence and your pre-baby body, and ensure your newborn is getting every ounce of vital nutrition he or she needs to grow into a healthy adult.

There are a variety of phases you and your child will go through during your lives, and each phase has a light at the end of the tunnel. Your experience and success in each phase depends on the decisions you choose and the lifestyle choices you make.

Come with me as I take you through each phase before, during, and after pregnancy. I'll share my tips and knowledge with you so your pregnancy will open up the door to a healthy, strong, and natural baby.

Chapter 1
Preconception: The Easy and the Hard Way

There are three types of individuals: the fertile, the non-fertile, and the in-between. Some women are blessed, and after one session of sex, the pee stick says "positive". Other women have to try a few times or for a few months or possibly even years, but eventually, it's "let's go buy some diapers!" Other women aren't so fortunate, and it is very difficult for them to conceive for many reasons. Possible reasons may include blocked fallopian tubes, irregular ovulation, too much stress and tension in their lives, problems with being over or underweight, ovarian cysts, or issues with a partner's sperm quality or count. However, there is still a slight chance for conception, no matter what the case may be.

Most fertility treatments nowadays are quite expensive and do not guarantee a 100% success rate. Having a healthy and well-balanced body may dramatically increase these chances. Even if you are one of those fortunate women who do not need to have medical assistance to conceive, but are still finding conception slow and difficult, a well-balanced body will dramatically increase your chances of becoming pregnant.

According to a 2008 landmark study based on the Harvard Nurses study, eating a wholefood, high plant-based diet with slow-release carbohydrates allows for a six-fold increase in fertility.

For those who were told you would never have a baby, please do not give up. Follow my guidelines and heal your body, reconstruct your thought pattern of negativity, and restore vitality in yourself. You may be surprised that with a positive attitude and a healthy, well-balanced body, conception may be a possibility after all – even if your chances are one in a million.

Preparing the mind and body

The first step really is to sit back and ask yourself how badly you want a baby. Do you want a child so much that you are willing to sacrifice those double lattes for breakfast and Friday night margaritas? Creating a balanced body is not, by any means, a diet of restriction, harsh cleansing, or expensive supplements. It is a lifestyle rich in healing, whole foods that are grown from the earth; foods that Mother Nature designed specifically for our health; foods that will help boost any woman's chance to conceive a baby.

If you have recently decided to have a baby and have been trying frequently but going nowhere, be patient and take the time to prepare your body for conception. Planning ahead is the wise choice at this moment. Before hopping upon the pregnancy bandwagon, gather your tools and start to build up your health and wellness. When you are at your best, it will be the best time to conceive.

The appropriate time to begin the healing and rebalancing of your body is approximately one year prior to trying to conceive. This gives both you and your partner plenty of time to allow your bodies to become strong and healthy before conceiving. Clearing your body of unwanted toxins that may be preventing you from becoming pregnant is your first goal. Through open-mindedness, positivity, and consistency, your chances of conception will dramatically increase and becoming pregnant will happen much easier.

Remember that you are not in this alone, and your partner should be following the same regime as you to rejuvenate his body and strengthen and increase his sperm count. Once the one-year mark is officially over, you can be ensured that you will be providing a safe, toxic-free environment for your baby with nothing but your powerful love and uterus surrounding it.

Take a deep breath and get ready for your complete body, mind, and soul makeover.

Vitamin A - 1st 8 weeks of pregnancy
- Bright fruits + vegetables
  - Oranges, Carrots, bell peppers, tomatoes, etc.
  - Beef, Chicken, Pork, Lamb

Vitamin C - Fruit
Vitamin D - Fat soluble vitamin - throughout pregnancy.
  - Supplements / sunshine
Vitamin E - Dark Leafy Greens + Avocados

B Vitamins - Red Meat, Chicken, Whole Grains
Folate - Green Leafy Vegetables, Asparagus, Broccoli
  - Absorbed best when cooked.

Biotin
Calcium
Iron   *Spinach, Red Meats, Chick Peas, beans

(omega 3,6,9)
Fish Oils - Fish Once a week
  - Cooking with Canola oil, Sunflower /safflower
  - Flax seeds / flax seed oil
  - Omega 3 eggs

- Mackerel   Stay away from: Tuna
- Talapia   Top-feeders
- Salmon

                    *(Inulin instead of glucose for test)
Sugar - Very little refined sugar

H₂O - lots of water

Power of digestion

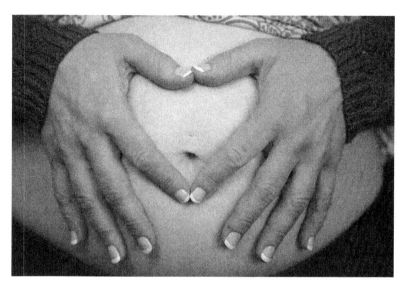

You come first photography

To begin your restoration of your health, you must begin by rebalancing the body and repairing one of the most essential body systems of all – the digestive system. The digestive system alone is responsible for 60 to 70 percent of your immunity. When the digestive system is ill, you are never fully well, and being well is a must for conception.

If your digestive system is not functioning optimally, your body will not be able to breakdown and absorb the nutrients needed for fertility and overall health. Toxins will begin to release themselves from the foods that were not fully digested and begin to cause illness, making it harder for all the body systems to optimally function.

Improper digestion can also lead to problems with elimination. If food cannot properly pass through our bodies, it again can build up unwanted toxins that can lead to illness.

The three main signs of a delay in the digestion system are bloating, gas, and constipation. A healthy digestion system will allow you to have at least one normal bowel movement a day. If constipation is an issue for you, your body is not breaking down food enough so it can easily pass through you. A high-fibre diet with plenty of water can help eliminate constipation without the use of stool softeners or laxatives.

The digestive system is also responsible for using the body's energy to digest the food consumed. If digestion is not properly functioning, it can use up over half of your daily energy output trying to break down food particles rather than rebalancing the rest of your body. Let's face it mamas, trying for a baby is no picnic in the park. It can be a tiring and lengthy process, so why not save up that much needed energy for sex rather than blow it all on digestion!

There are certain things you can do on a regular basis to promote healthy digestion:

1. **Do not drink with meals.** By consuming liquid at meal times, you are diluting the concentrated hydrochloric acid in the stomach, which is needed to properly break down and digest your food.

2. **Eat meals that contain animal products for dinner.** When we consume animal products such as chicken, beef, or seafood, these foods take much longer to pass through the digestive system and can even block other quicker digesting foods from passing though. This leads to fermentation and toxin production. My rule of thumb is to eat light to heavy: Lighter meals for breakfast and lunch and a heavier, more calorie-dense meal at supper. This allows for those easier-to-digest foods to be broken down efficiently, and then heavier foods have the entire night to be broken down before new food is reintroduced the next day at breakfast.

3. **Do not consume fruit with a meal that contains animal products.** As important as it is to consume meals with animal products in the evening, it is just as important to not consume fruit with these meals. Fruits are a simple carbohydrate which means the sugar contained in the fruit is digested the fastest. When combining these quick digesting sugars with slow digesting animal proteins, the fruit will begin to rot and ferment, which slows down digestion and causes symptoms such as gas and bloating.

4. **Eat a high plant-based diet.** Plant-based foods contain high amounts of fibre. Fibre is a complex carbohydrate that is indigestible by the body and is essential for digestive health. The different types of fibre – soluble and insoluble – contribute to sustaining regular bowel movements and maintaining a healthy colon. Fruits, vegetables, whole grains, and beans contain high amounts of fibre and should make up the majority of your diet. *In 2012, the Institute of Medicine recommended that adults should be consuming a minimum of 25 to 40 grams of fibre daily.* Unfortunately, the North American population consumes less than half of the recommended amount of daily fibre intake.

Balancing the system does take time and a bit of work, but can easily be done with the right tools, and you will learn these tools throughout my book. Once you've put the reins on digestion, all other systems of the body will begin to function more optimally as they are all tied into one. You will then begin to dramatically increase the amount of nutrients being absorbed into your body, excrete unwanted toxins, and focus on regaining homeostasis.

Food for thought

First is first. I always encourage my clients to start keeping a daily food journal for the first week or so. Logging each meal and beverage daily in complete detail will keep you accountable for knowing exactly what you're consuming on a daily basis.

This isn't about dramatically changing your lifestyle and food choices quite yet, but rather seeing where exactly you need to improve on your diet. Once your seven-day food log is completed, take a few minutes to thoroughly read it over and observe what you've consumed over that week. You might be surprised! It's quite amazing how studies have frequently found women consume more highly processed foods than they think.

Rather than constantly adding up calories for what you ate at breakfast, lunch, and dinner, focus on how much sugar, fat-filled, and processed foods you are consuming over all. It is just as important to observe all of the healthy food you are consuming in your diet. If the bad overpowers the good, then you must consider reassessing your food choices.

Creating a food log and noting every piece of food that goes into your mouth may seem like a waste of time, but it is an essential tool to stay organized and on track.

With all the good and bad food choices out there, it can be quite easy to misinterpret which foods are healthy and which are not. You may think you are eating a whole-foods diet when you're actually consuming many foods from the standard North American diet. Take a moment and really ask yourself if your grains are processed and refined or if they are whole grains. Are your fats coming from unhealthy sources such as red meat and butter? Or are they coming from avocados and coconut oil? These are all questions that can help change your thought patterns about how you eat. In the beginning, you are bound to have questions about if the food or the ingredients that you are consuming are in fact healthy for you.

What is really in your food?

This is where cleaning up your diet and focusing on healthy changes can get quite frustrating and confusing, especially when a product has more than one ingredient. My advice is to always seek help from labels and the list of ingredients on the back of a product. Reading labels for the list of ingredients is what will allow you to differentiate between the healthy and the unhealthy

Perhaps you are wondering about the muffin you ate for lunch. Was it indeed a healthy muffin because it was labelled "bran"? Or was it really just a baked concoction filled with processed flour, sugar, and chemicals? By simply looking at the back of the package, you will find everything you need to know right there in front of your eyes.

Labels can be deceiving, so always match the label with the ingredients. They easily go hand in hand. A bran muffin does sound quite healthy, as wheat bran contains plenty of fibre and is low in sugar. Unfortunately, the label does not tell you the exact volume of bran in the muffin. There could be 40 percent bran, and the remaining 60 percent of ingredients could be processed, which is usually the case with any store-bought baked goods. If the muffin has more then 10 grams of fat and over 30 grams of sugar, how can someone label that as a healthy muffin? Choose foods that are lower in fat and sugar with minimal to no processed ingredients.

grocery store can either be a horrible and confusing experience or a positive and easy experience, depending on how prepared you are. With numerous ingredients in a single product, you don't need to get overwhelmed. The secret of success is: If you cannot pronounce the ingredients, don't eat the product. Stay clear of any products with a laundry list of ingredients. Keep it simple by choosing products with very few ingredients as this can usually assure you that the product is not filled with toxic food additives. Choosing food products such as fresh fruits and vegetables will make grocery shopping much easier as these foods only contain one ingredient!

The "free" word

This is the word that is used in many diet products on the shelves of supermarkets. In fact, diet foods can be one of the most unhealthy food choices. They are usually filled with artificial ingredients to allow the food to be a lower calorie option without having to sacrifice the flavour or texture.

Avoid the "fat-free" and "sugar-free" labels!

Food marketers are the sneakiest bunch of them all. Products that are labelled fat-free and sugar-free are intended to make the eye see them as a healthy product that contains no sugar or fat. In general, this would be a healthy choice and most likely lower in calories. However, fat-free foods are usually loaded with sugar as the sugar replaces the lost flavour that the fat was providing before it was removed. Having a fat-free product with a massive amount of sugar prevents it from being a healthy product.

The same is true for sugar-free products. Yes, they may contain no fat AND no sugar, but they are most likely filled with artificial sweeteners. Sure your food now tastes super sweet without the added calories of real sugar, but you are now risking chemical exposure to your body and your infant. Choosing a lower fat version with no added sugar or a sugar-free product that uses a natural, zero-calorie sweetener such as stevia is your best choice.

The sugar effect

Numerous studies have shown a correlation between processed sugar consumption and decreased fertility rates. Sugar is the number one enemy to your body and your will power is the only line of defence to prevent this toxic compound from taking over.

Eating a diet high in refined sugars may negatively affect your chances of conception by causing a variety of problems within your body and conflicting with your body's natural homeostasis – aka balance. Overconsumption of this drug-like substance can cause:

1. Unbalanced hormones: Foods containing processed sugars are rapidly broken down by the body, which causes a rapid spike in blood sugars. When this occurs, the sugar spike reaches a climax or a temporary high that can last anywhere from 10 to 20 minutes. Our bodies crash once the high is over, leaving us feeling tired and drained. This occurs because during the crash period there is a constant stimulation of the adrenal glands as they try to replenish normal sugar levels by releasing the hormones cortisol and adrenaline. When are adrenal glands are continuously being over-stimulated, they eventually become sluggish and weak, which may lead to hormonal imbalances and a kink in the endocrine system. After a certain amount of continuous abuse of the adrenal glands, the hormones responsible for fertility – such as progesterone, estrogen, DHEA, and testosterone –can be affected.

2. The depletion of certain vitamins and minerals: When the body is forced to continuously produce generous amounts of insulin and cortisol, it starts to deplete certain stored vitamins and minerals in the body. These include vitamin E, magnesium, copper, and vitamin B6. Studies have shown that a body deficient in vitamin E can increase the chances of a miscarriage.

1. Insulin resistance: Every organ in your body plays an important role in your health. Your pancreas is the essential organ that secretes insulin to convert our blood sugar into food or energy for our cells. When we consume large amounts of sugar on a continuous basis, our pancreas is forced to produce large amounts of insulin. Over time, this can create an insulin resistance. Insulin resistance can contribute to abnormal ovulation by preventing ovulation or even affect the ability of the egg to implant in the uterus. Research has shown a major increase in miscarriages in woman who are insulin resistant.

Sugar is also an incredibly addictive substance. Studies have shown the effects of sugar on the body and mind are similar to the effects of cocaine. Sugar is also just as hard of an addiction to break as an addiction to cocaine.

So how do you know if you have a sugar addiction? How do you break free of it, and what is the effect on your body and the fetus? Detecting a sugar addiction can sometimes be difficult, as its symptoms can easily become part of your everyday life. Whether it is a serious addiction or not, breaking an addiction can be a real challenge. If you experience any of these symptoms, you may have a sugar addiction.

1. You have uncontrollable urges to eat unhealthy foods, even when you are truly not hungry.
2. You feel tired and heavy, especially after eating.
3. You are constantly thinking about sugar during the day until you satisfy your cravings with something sweet.

4. You get hormonal and have mood swings when you are not on a sugar high and eating something sugary balances your moods.

5. You have strong carbohydrate cravings for foods such as breads, pastas, and pastries.

Some people don't take having a sugar addiction seriously because they don't realize how serious it can actually become if it is not dealt with. Consuming too much sugar can lead to long-term consequences such as type two diabetes, obesity, tooth decay, chronic diseases, and an impaired immune system. It can also cause your baby to gain too much weight in the womb, which can lead to developing childhood obesity and diabetes in the future.

Although breaking a sugar addiction is quite difficult for most people, with some serious will power, it can be done. It's best to start off slowly and remove one to two sugary food items from your diet each week. This is similar to your pre-conception phase, when you slowly removed unhealthy food items from your diet each week to prevent over-indulgence.

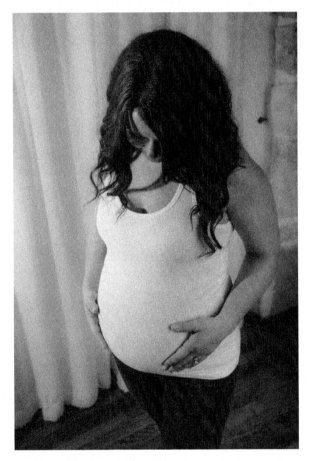

You come first photography

Follow these six tips to slowly wean yourself away from sugar and kick your addiction for good.

1. Eliminate soda, sweetened caffeinated beverages such as coffee or tea, juice (unless freshly pressed), and any other sugary beverages.

2. Eliminate candies, chocolate, baked goods, and other sugar-filled snacks and desserts.

3. Avoid processed carbs such as white breads, white pasta, pizza, and bleached flour. Replace these simple carbs with whole-grain, gluten-free versions.

4. Keep an eye out for hidden sugars. They can be everywhere from your ketchup or salad dressing to your tomato sauce and crackers. In today's society, sugar is in almost everything, so keep a close watch on prepackaged foods to ensure there is no added sugar.

5. Eat more fresh fruit! The sugar found in fruit is metabolized at a much slower rate than processed sugar. Fruit also has a ton of fibre, which stabilizes blood sugar and can keep you full.

6. Eat smaller meals and snacks throughout the day. Eating every 3 to 4 hours keeps your blood-sugar levels normal and prevents crashing and unexpected hunger. When you are hungry, sugar cravings kick in big time. Staying comfortably full throughout the day will prevent those cravings from happening. Eating every few hours also keeps the metabolism revving and your energy high.

Sugar by any other name

If you've ever looked at certain food products, especially products that would normally contain sugar such as cookies, cakes, and other baked goods, you may not see the word "sugar" in the ingredients. This does not mean that the product you're contemplating buying is healthy and contains no sugar.

The truth is that sugar can hide behind many names, even some that we would never expect to associate with sugar. To avoid sugar in disguise, you must learn the other terms that sugar can go by and make sure your product does not contain any of them.

Sugar/sucrose, which in its most popular form is known as table sugar or granulated sugar, comes from sugar cane or sugar beet plants. The juices of these plants are then extracted, crystallized, and processed into white sugar. Some natural products are sweetened with organic sugar cane, raw sugar, or evaporated cane juice, which is basically a less processed form of table sugar. However, it is still sugar and should be avoided as it contains 99 percent of sucrose, the main component in white sugar.

The following are three common, alterative names to sugar that are in numerous products. Be aware of these hidden sugars, and do your best to avoid products that contain them.

1. Brown sugar, which many people are convinced is much healthier than white sugar, is simply 95 percent sucrose and 5 percent molasses.

2. Fructose is a simple sugar that is naturally occurring in fruits and other foods. It is slightly sweeter than table sugar. You may notice that certain foods contain high fructose corn syrup, which is the processed and concentrated form of fructose. The fructose that is in fruit is metabolized much differently than the fructose in junk food and is actually healthy for you in moderate amounts.

3. Glucose/dextrose is the sugar that is produced from starches like potatoes. Again in its natural form, glucose is healthy for you as it is what feeds your brain and provides you with the energy you need to live. Glucose in products such as candy and other sweets is rapidly absorbed into the bloodstream and can stimulate a high insulin spike.

The following ingredients can also camouflage sugar:
- Tapioca syrup
- Barley malt
- Beet sugar
- Caramel
- Corn syrup
- Fruit juice concentrates
- Pasteurized honey
- Malt syrup
- Lactose
- Maltodextrin

Fortunately, there are natural sweeteners that hold certain health properties and have a much lower glycemic index than sugar.

My top six sweeteners are a much better choice than processed sugar:

1. Agave nectar (also known as agave syrup) is a natural sweetener that is made from the agave plant. It contains higher levels of fructose than other natural sweeteners, so it should be used in moderation. Best uses: Baking

2. Stevia is a zero-calorie sweetener that is extracted from the leaves of the stevia plant. Best uses: Baking, coffee/tea, salad dressings, smoothies, and other beverages

3. Brown rice syrup is a thick syrup made from rice starch. It contains high levels of B vitamins. Best uses: Pancakes/waffles, toast

4. Coconut palm sugar is a caramel, brown-sugar-like sweetener that is produced from the nectar of coconut palm trees. Best uses: Baking, coffee/tea

5. Xylitol is a naturally occurring sweetener that is extracted from many of the fruits and vegetables we consume. It is also calorie free. Best uses: Baking, coffee/tea, drinks, salad dressings, smoothies, and other beverages

6. Raw, unpasteurized honey is a delicious, sweet-tasting syrup made from our friends the bees by using the nectar from flowers. Do not confuse raw honey with the traditional pasteurized honey, which has been heated to extreme temperatures and is much less nutrient dense. Best uses: Baking, pancakes/waffles, toast, tea, and smoothies

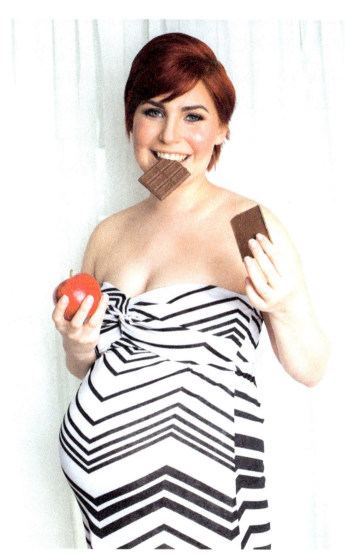

You come first photography

To be or not to be organic?

Eating organic foods should be one of the top priorities for expectant mothers, and I will explain why. When doing your grocery shopping, aim to purchase organic foods as much as possible, as this will benefit you and your baby much more than the generic, non-organic foods. Today's society sometimes questions whether or not the whole organic ideal is actually worth it or not. The truth is that it most definitely is. When a product is labelled organic, it is stating that the food was grown without the use of pesticides and insecticides.

Organic produce is also grown in nutrient-rich soil, which gives more nutrients to the organic food than if it were grown in standard soil as most produce is today. It is extremely important to avoid foods that contain these harsh chemicals, pesticides, and insecticides when trying to conceive. It is also just as important that your partner removes these additives from his diet.

A number of pesticides have been associated with impaired fertility in males. Mothers who consume these harsh substances while pregnant or trying to conceive have an increased chance of experiencing altered fetal growth, having babies born with birth defects, and even deliver a stillborn. By consuming inorganic products, you are ingesting the particles responsible for some cancers (such as brain, breast, skin, and liver cancer), as well as illnesses like depression and even dementia. In addition to affecting yourself, your unborn child could suffer even more from chemical exposure.

Many individuals think that if you wash your fruit and vegetables you will not have to worry about ingesting these toxins. Wrong! When pesticides are sprayed on fruits and vegetables, the pesticides are actually absorbed into the food, leaving harmful trace residues. Therefore, washing your produce will not guarantee a 100% removal of pesticides.

Mamas, this is your chance for conceiving and growing a healthy baby by consuming an organic diet. Another positive aspect of eating organic produce is that there is scientific evidence that organic fruits and vegetables have a higher amount of vitamins due to the fragile and uncontaminated soil in which they are grown. *For instance, a 2003 study in* the Journal of Agricultural and Food Chemistry *found that organically grown berries and corn contained 58 percent more polyphenols – antioxidants that help prevent cardiovascular disease – and up to 52 percent higher levels of vitamin C than those conventionally grown.* (http://www.eatingwell.com).

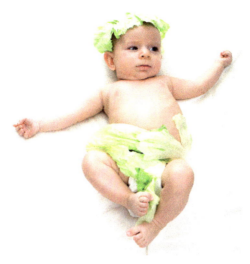

You come first photography

Realistically, not everyone can afford to only buy organic food, as it does cost slightly more than non-organic. Do your best to purchase what you can afford and focus on the foods that are most at risk for chemical exposure.

The dirty dozen

The dirty dozen list of produce was invented to show the consumer the most important kinds of organic produce to purchase. Some foods can get away without being organically grown as they have less exposure to pesticides, while other kinds of produce have a higher exposure.

The following foods should only be purchased if they are organically grown. If you cannot find one of these items labelled organic, it is highly recommended you find an alternative.

1. Apples
2. Blueberries
3. Grapes
4. Celery
5. Peaches
6. Spinach
7. Bell peppers

8. Nectarines
9. Tomatoes
10. Snap peas
11. Potatoes
12. Lettuce

A gentle detox

Let's help prepare our bodies not only by removing the fatty, processed, and high sugar foods, but also by removing the hidden additives as well. It is extremely important to take this process slowly. By ridding the body of toxins too quickly, you are risking your body going into detox mode and releasing too many toxins back into your circulatory system. This can cause your body's elimination systems to become overloaded. Having your body detox too quickly may cause unwanted symptoms such as illness, acne, stomach aches, headaches, minor depression, respiratory problems, and more.

Take it one step at a time, slowly replacing processed foods with whole food choices until your entire diet is unprocessed. If your current way of eating is already quite clean and free from toxic food, you should be more than okay to go full throttle on cleaning up your diet and removing all processed foods. Detoxing too quickly can also result in a whiplash of unwanted cravings, leading to an episode of binge eating – which none of us want.

With all the different foods sitting around on the store shelves, it may be hard at first to avoid every single unhealthy choice. In terms of pregnancy and good health in general, there are three products that should be completely avoided. These foods can increase the risk of developing illness.

1. Diet soda: Although considered safe for human consumption by the FDA when it was approved in 1974, the chemicals and artificial ingredients in these beverages are certainly not. In particular, I am pointing at the main one that contributes to the sweetness of these drinks. That culprit is aspartame. I speak more about aspartame later on in my book when talking about food additives to avoid. It is a dangerous product to ingest, especially when trying to conceive. Studies show that aspartame contributes to brain damage in those who drink it on a continuous basis. A study on rats was done that showed tumours in the brains of rats that were given aspartame. This took it off the market until 1981, when it was again approved. Even if a product is listed as safe, it does not mean that there are no hidden side effects and long-term consequences that can come from it. If you are seriously considering trying to conceive, this is on the top of my list of dangerous food additives you MUST avoid!

2. Dairy: Ah, good old dairy. We hear how it's filled with calcium and vitamin D, it's great for the bones to prevent osteoporosis, and it's filled with many other health benefits. It is listed on the Canadian Food Guide as a "food group"! It can also be what is making us extremely sick.

First, I'd like to try and help you all realize why we are NOT meant to digest dairy. When a human being is born, that human relies on his/her mother's milk in order to grow and survive until he/she is old enough to eat solid foods. At that point, the baby no longer requires breast milk. So why would a baby drink the milk from another mammal? You never see a newborn calf drinking from the breast of another animal do you? (Of course there are certain circumstances where a baby animal is supplemented with another animal's milk to increase its chances of survival.) That is because the bodies of all mammals are designed to drink only the milk of their kind. Cow's milk is perfectly designed for calves as it contains every nutrient they specifically need.

So why is it that as adults, we drink breast milk from an animal? Sounds a bit odd when you think of it like that, right? A baby's only food for the first 6 months is milk, and when they are mature enough, solid foods are introduced into their diet. But we are far older than 6 months, and we are drinking the milk from a species other than our own. It would make so much more sense if adults drank human breast milk every day instead of a cow's breast milk! But we do not.

We drink a substance designed for a calf. This makes the body wonder what the substance is. Some of us can easily digest dairy, but others are sensitive to it or are lactose intolerant. This occurs when a body is lacking the enzyme lactase, which is needed to help break down the sugar found in milk called lactose. The enzyme is a main component in breast milk, making it easily digested by babies since they are getting this enzyme through the mother's milk. However, as we age, our ability to produce this enzyme starts to decrease, since we are no longer nursing from our mothers. This can cause our digestive systems to react poorly to the lactose in milk.

Diary is foreign to our "natural design", which is why it is difficult to digest and can lead to an abundance of other health problems. Dairy products are also very acidic to the body. The human body is meant to be in a slightly alkaline state. We are meant to believe that drinking dairy benefits our bones by making them stronger, when it really does the opposite. In order to neutralize the acidity in your body caused by the continuous consumption of dairy products, your body will start to draw calcium and phosphorus from your bones to bring the body back to its natural alkaline state.

According to Dr. Amy Lanou, Nutrition Director for the Physicians Committee for Responsible Medicine in Washington, D.C., "The countries with the highest rates of osteoporosis are the ones where people drink the most milk and have the most calcium in their diets. The connection between calcium consumption and bone health is actually very weak, and the connection between dairy consumption and bone health is almost nonexistent."

Dairy, if not organic, actually contains harmful ingredients such as hormones, antibiotics, and chemicals to help ensure the cows stay healthy, grow strong, avoid illness, and continue to produce a large amount of milk. Unfortunately, the harmful additives that are given to cows throughout their life are absorbed and transferred to their milk. These are then absorbed into our bodies when we consume dairy. These additives can be a huge cause for infertility. In simpler terms: Avoid dairy at all cost! Dairy is the perfect food for a calf! If you absolutely must have a piece of cheese or glass of milk, opt for organic, unpasteurized goat cheese or milk. It is much easier for the body to digest.

3. Gluten: This is the protein composition of wheat and other related grains. Gluten, comes from the Latin world "glue", which says it all. When gluten begins to digest in the body, it forms a glue-like substance that is very difficult for the body to digest. This is why gluten allergies are on the rise and are so commonly found in individuals today. Making sure your food is easily digestible is very important when it comes to fertility.

You are probably turning to your partner at this moment saying, "I can never eat bread or pasta again?" That is not the case. You can still enjoy all of your favourite foods by replacing them with a gluten-free alternative. Get creative with a variety of different grains and see what your cravings can come up with!

Top gluten-free grains:
- Gluten-free brown rice or organic corn pasta
- Gluten-free breads, wraps, and other baked goods
- Brown and wild rice
- Quinoa
- Amaranth
- Buckwheat
- Corn (make sure it comes from non-GMO crops and be careful as corn is a common food allergy for some)
- Millet
- Gluten-free oats
- Teff

If you notice symptoms such as constipation, gas, bloating, hives, headaches, pain in your gut (especially after eating), fatigue, rashes, dandruff, depression, and irritability, you may have a gluten sensitivity. Whether or not you are gluten sensitive, it is still wise to draw out all food products with gluten from your diet for the sake of your digestion, fertility, and overall health.

Ride the whole foods wave

With the removal of so many unhealthy foods (such as gluten and dairy) from your diet, you may be worrying that you are not taking in a sufficient amount of calories to sustain yourself and all your daily activities. This is not the case. As long as you are replacing the processed and refined foods you were consuming on a regular basis with healthy alternatives made from whole foods, you will be getting plenty of healthy calories to keep you energetic and on the go. You may also be surprised to notice an increase in energy and well-being once you start consuming a diet of whole, unprocessed foods. These feelings are brought on when the body has flushed out the majority of toxins that it has built up over time. Your body is no longer an old car running on dirty oil and low fuel. It's a much newer model running on clean oil and a full tank!

Its important to understand that this way of eating is a lifestyle change and not just a quick fix diet, so patience is a must. You may still be consuming a few meals a week that are not considered to be part of this lifestyle change, but you are still reaping the benefits of detoxing your body. Continue to remove the unhealthy meals weekly and you will notice your whole diet has transformed within a couple of months. It will eventually become second nature to you, and eating clean will be a part of your daily regime. Just listen to your body and do what feels right.

It's not at all difficult to begin the transition to eating a whole foods diet. You can easily find healthy alternatives to what you eat on a regular basis. For example: Substitute generic, fatty, fried eggs with organic, free-range, hard-boiled eggs. Rather than choose the white toast with butter, opt for a slice of whole-grain, gluten-free toast with some sliced avocado and tomato. Just by doing these simple swaps with most or all of your meals, you will have removed at least 80-90% of unhealthy fats and processed food products from your diet. At the same time, you will also be adding an abundance of nutrients like fibre and vitamin C.

Keep with this regime for as long as you can. Remember, you are preparing a year ahead for your baby, so you may be tempted now and then to slip back into your old ways. Just make sure you keep things interesting. Always keep a variety of whole food items around so you are not stuck eating the same meals day after day. Spice up your meals with some fresh sea salt, or better yet, pink Himalayan salt found at your local health store. Try adding some peppers and even some spices with no added salt. (Mrs. Dash is great or opt for an organic spice.) Some spices like the Indian spice Shatavari, is actually used by women to improve fertility and stimulate sexuality.

After regularly eating a whole-food diet, or even if you have just recently started, you may notice that you begin to have cravings for your old foods. Unfortunately, this is common. The good news is that there are tricks and tips you can do to avoid slipping back into your old eating habits. One great way to stick to your healthy lifestyle is to create a healthy version of your craving. If you really miss those delicious, barbequed hamburgers you used to enjoy every weekend, you don't have to skip out on those bad boys. Instead, remake them by removing the typical fatty and processed ingredients and replacing them with a healthier version. Go to the market and buy some organic (if possible) ground, extra-lean turkey breast. Chop up some onion and bell peppers, and form into patties. Put on the barbecue and grill. Put these burgers on a gluten-free bun, or better yet, add some romaine lettuce cups with tomato, pickles, and any other veggies you fancy, and a little Dijon mustard, and there you have it. You might not even want to go back to your old greasy burgers ever again.

If you do happen to run into a wall and opt for some of your old treats, don't hate yourself and feel guilty. Have what you need and leave the rest alone. The key is to try to not go overboard when indulging. There is a reason why we call it an indulgence, rather than a binge. A small amount of an unhealthy food once in a while will not throw your whole lifestyle change out the window. After your indulgence, start fresh the next meal. Having your favourite treats once in a while and eating them only in moderation will help keep you on the track to conception! Don't forget that there are also plenty of delicious alternatives, sweet and salty, that are easy to whip up as replacements for your favourite munchies. Later in my book, I share with you a several of my recipes to keep you from reaching into the cookie jar!

At this point, you and your partner are learning the concepts of healthy eating and are well on your way to cleaning up your current eating habits. Keep in mind that if you fall off the baby wagon, you can get right back on it! Tomorrow is brand new day and a new time to begin putting clean, whole foods back in your body.

Chapter 2
"F" Is for Fertility

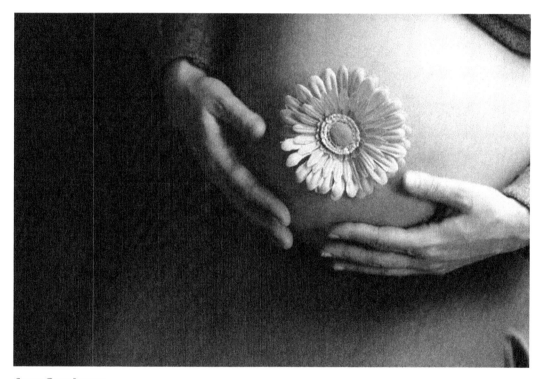

Sweet Grass Images

Fertility food and what to watch out for

Many researchers today have found various foods that can help increase the chances of conception and positively affect fertility in both males and females. It isn't just about eating organic, even though that is one of the most important aspects in holistic nutrition. It is also about the types of foods you should consume more of and others you should avoid completely, as there are some products that can have a negative effect on fertility.

With all the packaged foods in today's society, there are certain processed foods that actually hold sufficient nutrient value.

Healthy and not-so-healthy packaged foods

The majority of packaged food on the market today is unfortunately the unhealthy kind. However, hidden in the aisles of the grocery store, you will stumble upon certain packaged foods that are in fact good for you. Although healthy packaged foods may go through somewhat of a process in order to become a product like sprouted grain bread or whole-grain cereal, they do not usually contain any harmful ingredients and have not suffered from a great amount of nutrient loss.

If buying packaged foods, seek out the products made from whole foods, such as gluten-free pasta, wild rice, and quinoa. These products consist generally of whole food ingredients and are free of any artificial preservatives.

Prepackaged foods to avoid are items such as macaroni and cheese, canned vegetables, overly salted soups, frozen entrees, chips, doughnuts, cookies, candy, and well, everything that has more than a few ingredients listed. These foods are filled with large amounts of sodium, processed and refined carbohydrates, sugar, and saturated and trans fats. Aim for fresh meals you can prepare at home or packaged, whole food meals.

The lowdown on food additives

If you are planning on purchasing prepackaged foods, be aware of the food additives that can actually cause serious damage to your body and have a negative impact on your fetus.

MSG: Monosodium glutamate (MSG) is actually the salt of the amino acid glutamate. It acts as a flavour enhancer to bring out the best flavours in foods. It is commonly found in Chinese food, canned veggies, processed meats, and soups. Although the FDA considers MSG to be relatively safe, it has been known to cause common symptoms in many individuals such as: headaches, flushing, nausea, chest pain, and heart palpitations. It is best to avoid this ingredient, mamas-to-be and current mamas, as it can affect your body in a negative way, as well as affect your baby. Recent studies have shown that MSG when broken down into something called "free glutamates" can actually cross through the placenta barrier. If there are too many free glutamates for your body to handle, your baby will absorb the excess that is circulating in your body through your bloodstream. MSG has also been known to cause bran cell injuries in baby mice, so we are just better off without those three letters on our plates.

BHT and BHA: These are antioxidants commonly used as preservatives. These additives can cause allergic reactions and even cancer when stored in the body. Common foods containing BHT and BHA are cereals, canned legumes, and potato chips.

Food colourings, including tartrazine: Because there is not a lot of testing done of food colourings to ensure they are safe for our consumption, it is best to avoid them. There has also been research done that indicates they can be carcinogens (cancer causing) and increase hyperactivity. These food colourings can be found in almost any processed food, especially CANDY! Check your labels, moms, or better yet, opt for organic candy or dried fruit (without sulfites) to satisfy your sweet tooth. Organic candies never have those artificial ingredients and are often coloured with beet juice and other fruit and veggie complexes.

Aspartame: Ah! This artificial sweetener is found in almost anything sugar-free (except for products using Splenda) and is also a NO-NO. Aspartame is known to cause brain damage in individuals when consumed on a constant basis. If you are really in the mood for a fizzy, sweet drink, opt for sparkling juice or soda water with lime or cranberry.

Caffeine: It is wise to limit your caffeine intake during pregnancy to no more then two small cups of coffee or caffeinated tea a day. It is even better to completely remove caffeinated products from your diet when you are trying to conceive and while pregnant. Overconsumption of caffeine while pregnant can cause birth defects and even miscarriages. Caffeine today is found in many other beverages and some food products besides tea and coffee. It is found in soda and CHOCOLATE! Don't worry ladies; still enjoy your chocolate, just in moderation.

Sulfites, nitrates, and sodium nitrates: These are cancer-causing chemicals found in today's processed foods such as bacon, lunch/deli meats, and hot dogs. Stay clear of these foods while pregnant as they can be very harmful to the baby.

Non-organic dairy and animal products: (I recommend excluding all dairy from your diet, but if you do have small amounts, be sure it is organic or try a dairy alternative such as unsweetened almond or hemp milk.) Diary and animal products that are not labelled organic are usually injected with a growth hormone called "bovine". This hormone is used to help cows produce more milk and to increase the growth of animals used for slaughter. These animals are also injected with many antibiotics to prevent sickness from occurring and spreading amongst the herd. These hormones and antibiotics have been reported to cause early puberty in girls, resulting in a higher chance of breast and other forms of cancer in their future. We as future or current parents want to ensure that we are staying clear of these hormones and antibiotics. It is almost as bad as injecting your newborn with drugs and prescriptions and not knowing the side effects. Opt for organic, and you'll have a much better chance at obtaining good health.

While avoiding these harmful chemicals and food additives, you are ensuring the safety of yourself and your fetus. Ladies who are having problems with conceiving should pay close attention to ensure that any dairy or animal products they consume are 100% organic and hormone-free. These chemicals can interfere with your fertility and dramatically decrease your chances of conceiving.

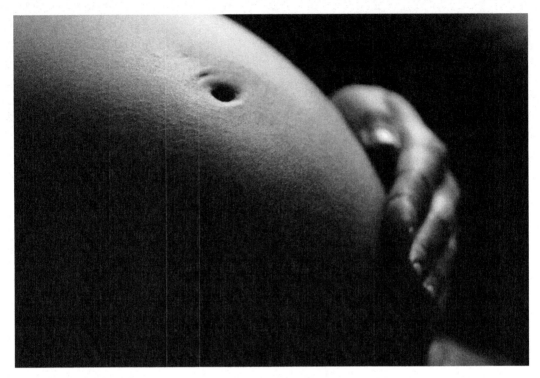

Sweet Grass Images

Supplementations

Now that the food part has been covered, it's time to move on to another crucial aspect of fertility – that is, supplements. There are many supplements on the market today – whether synthetic, natural, good or bad, vitamins or minerals. The good quality ones can play a large part in increasing fertility in both men and women.

If you ever go to a pharmacy or natural food store and look on the shelves, you will notice the hundreds of different supplements and brands out there today on the market. But which one should you choose? There is everything from solid pills and capsules to liquids, chewables, and powders. It can be confusing. When choosing the right supplements, you want to consider a few things. If you have a bad digestive system where your body takes longer to digest or lacks the production of hydrochloric acid, you may not be getting the most out of your vitamins. The longer a supplement takes to dissolve, the fewer the nutrients that are actually being absorbed. Instead they are being diluted while waiting to be digested by your body. The best form of supplements to consume to ensure you are absorbing 95-100% of the nutrients are powders and liquids. These are easily broken down by the digestive system and quickly absorbed by the body.

Synthetic vs. Natural

Once you have found which supplement form is right for you, it is time to do a little research to determine whether your supplement is natural or artificial. All you have to do is look at the label on the bottle, and it should be listed as "natural" or "synthetic". Natural supplements are produced from natural sources such as extracts from fruits and veggies. In other words, they are from whole foods. Synthetic supplements do not perform the same functions in your body as the natural ones. Synthetic supplements can actually deplete the body of other vital nutrients. Natural is always the way to go, and if you can locate natural supplements deprived from organic whole foods, that is even better. To find the highest quality vitamins and minerals, drive to your nearest health food store. Their selection is almost always natural and comes from organic food sources.

The magic pill

Prenatal vitamins are a great way to kick-start fertility. They contain higher amounts of the essential vitamins and minerals than the typical adult multivitamin. They also contain a very important vitamin called Foliate or vitamin B9, which can contribute to your chances of conception. Taking at least 400 micrograms of folic acid a day reduces the risk of neural tube defects by up to 70%. To add to your folic acid intake, there are many additional foods you can consume such as leafy green vegetables, kidney beans, orange juice and other citrus fruits, peanuts, broccoli, asparagus, peas, lentils, and whole-grain products.

Prenatal vitamins also contain important nutrients and antioxidants such as vitamin C, zinc, and vitamin E, along with many other essential nutrients to provide everything you and baby will need. Do not just rely on supplements alone; nothing can make up for a diet full of variety and healthy, whole foods. Pair your current healthy diet with a high-quality prenatal vitamin and you are good to go!

C is for conception

Although your prenatal vitamin already has a good amount of vitamin C, taking an extra vitamin C supplement (1000 mg a day) is recommended to aid in fertility. If you do not wish to take an additional vitamin C supplement, there are plenty of foods that contain vitamin C – such as citrus fruits and juices, red or yellow peppers, and broccoli.

Your supplements are best taken in the morning with your breakfast. To really maximize the fertility-boosting affects of a healthy diet, be sure to include many colourful fruits and veggies with a variety of whole grains and lean protein throughout the day. You will benefit much more by mixing up your food choices, rather than eating the same foods daily. Add some colour to your meals or even try a new healthy food you have never tasted before!

The miraculous plant

There are many natural herbal supplements on the market today that aid fertility and healthy pregnancies. Through my research, I have come across one supplement, which I have tried myself and found to help in maintaining a healthy pregnancy. Maca is a nourishing food for the endocrine system and aids the pituitary, thyroid, and adrenal glands. These glands are responsible for creating and balancing hormones. Maca actually works by helping to stimulate and nourish the pituitary gland and allowing it to function normally. When the pituitary is functioning properly, it balances out the entire endocrine system. Balancing the hormones and keeping their levels at bay is a major contributor to a healthy body. Women produce the hormone estrogen. When estrogen levels are too high or too low, it may prevent a woman from carrying to term. Supplementing with maca can actually balance out estrogen levels in the body, increasing the chances of having a healthy, full-term pregnancy.

Exercise and alternative medicine

Women who are obese or have a high Body Max Index (BMI) have a lesser chance of conceiving than those of a healthy weight. It is best to get and keep your BMI between 18.5 and 25. There are many online calculators, which will calculate your BMI and give you a good idea if you need to increase your workouts! It is important that while you are trying to conceive, you do at least 30 minutes of low- to medium-intensity physical activity at least 3 to 5 times a day. Talking a brisk walk for half an hour every day will give your body the head start it needs to get prepared for baby. Being active on a daily basis helps increase blood flow to the body, reduce stress and body fat, and keep your heart healthy. All of these will help in maintaining your health and weight when trying to conceive.

Traditional Chinese medicine

Traditional Chinese medicine can help naturally optimize your fertility. Getting acupuncture treatment approximately 4 to 6 months before conception is a good timeline to abide by. Many holistic practitioners describe the human body as an energy field and the female reproductive system as a network in the energy field. Having unbalanced body energy is believed to have negative effects on your reproductive system. These imbalances can be caused by stress, poor diet, lack of exercise, and environmental chemicals. A traditional Chinese medicine practitioner will point out your imbalances and perform effective acupuncture treatments, as well as provide you with a customized herb program to help rebalance your body's systems and increase your chances of fertility and pregnancy. Acupuncture will help reduce stress, which can effect a person's health dramatically. It can encourage relaxation, strengthen the immune system, regulate hormones, and improve sperm count in males. Because traditional Chinese medicine has been around for many years, it has been proven that these treatments can be very beneficial.

Visit the chiropractor

Chiropractic care is a safe and natural approach to enhancing the body's ability to function properly. This is accomplished through enhancing the body's nervous system.

How might cracking bones and realigning the body benefit a woman's fertility, you may ask? In many cases, fertility problems may be associated with improper functioning of the nervous system, unhealthy nutrition, high stress, and poor lifestyle habits. Chiropractors are actually nervous system specialists who work by reducing interference in the nervous system. Their efforts keep the spine properly aligned, help balance out the body, and allow the nervous system to function properly. Chiropractors are one of your best options to help your body function in harmony with the way it was designed.

See a nutritionist

Yes, there are dieticians, nutritionists, and food coaches all across the world. But the one person who knows more about whole and natural foods and how to use these foods to re-balance the body in a healthy way is a holistic nutritionist. A holistic nutritionist is a health care professional trained in natural nutrition and to determine the cause of ill health and correct it using natural whole foods, and supplements. Their principal function is to educate individuals about the benefits and health impact of optimal nutrition.

Many holistic nutritionists have experience working with women having trouble conceiving. Customized meal and supplementation plans can be designed to teach these women about certain foods they should avoid or increase in order to heal their body and increase their chances of fertility.

They will also recommend which supplements can be taken along with a proper diet to further increase the chances of fertility. Book an appointment with a holistic nutritionist who has previous experience with prenatal clients to ensure you are getting the best knowledge and support.

Chapter 3
What You Need to Know in Your First Trimester

Honey, I'm pregnant!

Congratulations! You are officially a mom-to-be. And for those who have a little more trying to do, continue keeping yourself healthy, stress-free, and in a confident mind frame. Your time is coming. There is no exact timeline, as each woman is different, and some may need more time to prep. They key is to stay positive and don't give up. For those who have become pregnant, you will now experience many new changes over the next 9 months. You are beautiful woman who has provided her baby with a safe, healthy, and non-toxic environment in which to grow and become strong as it makes its way into the world.

You have taken care of your body for a whole year (some more, some less). You have worshipped it and given it the vital nutrients of survival and ultimate health. You have healed most or all of your imbalances and have prepared for the journey of pregnancy. Keep in mind that even though you are now pregnant and your time of trying to conceive has come to an end, your healthy body and natural lifestyle have not. You must continue now to eat healthy, whole, natural foods; replenish your body with the fluids of the earth; and supplement with high-quality vitamins and minerals. This will not just benefit you as an expectant mother, but also your future child you are carrying inside you.

This is the time in your life where you begin to put your child first. Whatever you give to yourself, you are giving to your baby. Provide yourself with nourishment and happiness, relaxation and peace, and you will be providing your unborn baby with the same nurturing care. This love you have for yourself ensures that your baby will have a happy, stress-free journey in your womb, and come into the world the same way. A baby who is born with little to no stress and into a stress-free environment suffers from less illness and emotional problems as it grows in comparison to a baby who has gone through a stressful 9 months of pregnancy as well as a traumatic birth. This child is already predetermined to have a more stressful life. Giving birth to a calm child means you will find it easier to put your baby to sleep and to feed it, and your child will have less fussing and health concerns.

So what is next? Who do you need to see and what do you need to do now that you are pregnant? There is one main answer: Listen to your body. Eat when you are hungry. Stop when you are full. Rest when you need it, and stay active when you are energetic. Never force your body into doing something it does not want to do. You will also want to contact a health provider as soon as possible, as they will assist you in your journey through pregnancy, birth, and post partum.

Midwife or doctor?

Having a midwife to look after yourself and your unborn baby may be a lot less stressful than being taken care of by a medical doctor. Not to say that doctors are not professionals and reliable for providing you with the best advice and care through your 9-month journey. But if you choose to take a more natural approach, a midwife may be the better choice.

Most of the care that midwives provide is in the community, creating significant savings for the health care system. This results in a high rate of client satisfaction and significantly reduces the demand for hospital services. By being on-call around the clock for their clients, midwives reduce ER visits. As well, one in four clients give birth at home. Women who give birth in the hospital with a midwife have shorter hospital stays, lower re-admission rates, and lower obstetrical intervention rates. So if you are planning to give birth at home or without any induction and/or pain medication, consider a midwife over a clinical doctor.

Need a bit of extra support? Consider hiring a doula!

A doula is an individual who provides support for a woman and her partner before or after childbirth. Although doulas are not covered by health insurance, many mothers appreciate the extra physical and emotional support. Doulas can relieve many stressors during the time of labour from getting food and drinks to ensuring the doctor and nurses are aware of the mother's birthing plan. They also provide wonderful assistance in comforting the mother with different relaxation techniques in the early stages of labour.

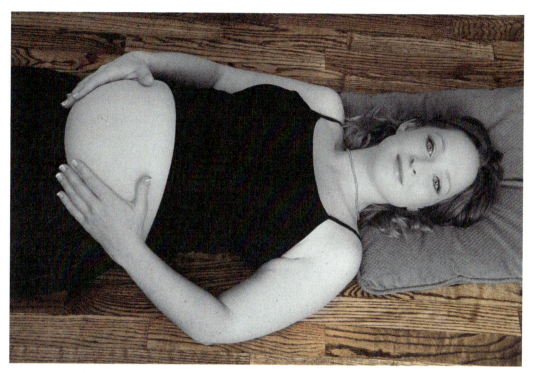

You come first photography

The reality

The first trimester is one of the most important trimesters throughout pregnancy, as this is when most of your baby's critical developmental takes place. It is extremely important to practice good health and nutrition during this stage and make sure you continue to take your prenatal vitamins throughout your whole pregnancy. There are certain nutrients required in the three stages of pregnancy, and you must ensure you are getting the recommended amounts.

During this phase of pregnancy, you are not required to up your calorie intake as the fetus is quite small and can obtain all the nutrients it needs through your normal eating habits. You are required to gain only 1 to 5 pounds(0.5-2.2 kg) in the first trimester. An average weight gain during an entire pregnancy is anywhere from 25 to 35 pounds (11-15 kg). For an underweight woman it might be roughly 28 to 40 pounds(12-18 kg), and for an overweight woman the weight gain should be no more than 15 to 20 pounds(6-9 kg).

Being pregnant and needing a caloric increase does not give you permission to indulge in ice cream and chocolate bars for breakfast. The majority of mothers assume that during this time they are allowed to eat whatever they would like. I highly recommend removing yourself from this stereotype and sticking to a whole foods diet with minimal indulgences. Sure, you're bound to have strong cravings that can sometimes become very overwhelming. It's perfectly acceptable to give in to these cravings, as long as you do it in moderation. Balance is the key to having a healthy pregnancy.

Unfortunately, as many as 75 percent of expectant mothers get morning sickness. Nausea and vomiting can eventually cause some weight loss. Don't be alarmed if it's just a few pounds, but if you notice yourself losing large amounts of weight or are unable to keep any food or liquids down, seek medical attention immediately.

Morning sickness: Am I supposed to feel like this?

Here is the straight up truth: In your first trimester you will likely feel horrible – at least for most moms. Only a small percent of expectant mothers are the fortunate ones who do not experience any pregnancy symptoms. If you are one of those fortunate ones, continue to do your thing! Moms who aren't so fortunate may feel mild to harsh symptoms of fatigue, nausea, morning sickness, headaches, constipation, sleep disorders, etc. These symptoms are completely normal and likely will go away in the second trimester. However, they may come back in your third semester, so take advantage when you can.

For those who are suffering from constant morning sickness and nausea, it is still very important to eat healthy and stay hydrated. For myself personally, the only thing I could stomach for the first four months of my pregnancy was fruit and sandwiches. There are some moms who only crave cookies and ice cream, others who crave greens and veggies, and some mothers who simply cannot hold anything down. As hard is it may be to consume those healthy, whole foods when your body simply does not want them, it is still necessary as your body needs those vital nutrients for your baby.

Dark green, leafy vegetables should be the most consumed food in your pregnancy diet as they are very nutrient dense and contain the highest amount of vitamins and minerals your body needs. Consuming these greens while feeling sick may be very difficult, but there are some ways to sneak them into your daily meals.

Throwing some spinach or kale in with your morning smoothie is a great way to get in those essential greens. The fruit camouflages the taste of any greens so it will be an easy way to get them into your diet. Blending your fruits and vegetables will make the meal more easily digestible so you are able to absorb its nutrients more efficiently.

Can't stomach the smoothie? Consider supplementing your diet with a concentrated greens powder. Greens powder is basically a compound of mixed greens and super foods that have been ground down into a fine powder. It is packed with essential vitamins and minerals and can provide you with a needed energy boost. The powders usually come flavoured and unflavoured, so you can choose either option depending on your taste. Simply mix with some filtered water or fresh juice and enjoy. Greens powders can be purchased from any health store.

Feeling unwell during pregnancy is most certainly unpleasant and is more severe than feeling nauseated from a common cold or flu. If you are constantly throwing up, your body will not be able to absorb sufficient nutrients, and more importantly, it will be much harder to stay hydrated.

If you are suffering from morning sickness, it's absolutely crucial to drink water, and lots of it. The human body is made up 60% water, and let's not forget the extra water your amniotic fluid contains. While you are pregnant, your blood volume also increases a whopping 45%, and water is necessary for this to happen. A lack of water during pregnancy can cause even more fatigue, nausea, and irritation – even if you are only slightly dehydrated. If you are severely dehydrated, it can cause the blood fluid levels to deplete and make you more prone to bladder infections. Ouch! As you progress in pregnancy, dehydration can even cause you to go into premature labour by triggering contractions, and that is something you definitely don't want.

Some mothers find they cannot stomach plain water. With other alternatives it is easy to find a healthy and delicious beverage you will enjoy that will still provide you with hydration and heath benefits. The following are some alternatives to water:

> Flavoured water: Simply adding some fresh lemon, orange, or lime juice to your water can alter the flavour of your beverage and make it more drinkable. You can also try slicing a small piece of fresh ginger and allowing it to soak in a bottle of water for a few hours. The strong flavours of the ginger will be absorbed into the water, making it easier to get down. In addition, ginger can help to decrease nausea.

> Coconut water: This is an all-natural beverage that comes from young coconuts. They are not old enough to contain milk; so instead, you get a clear liquid filled with vital nutrients that support natural hydration. Also the sweet taste of coconuts can be very easy to drink and can even help settle the stomach. With it containing natural sugars, electrolytes, and potassium, you are getting a balance of nutrients that is good for you and your baby. It is even a great energy booster when you're feeling a bit sluggish. The natural sugars will give you just enough of a push without causing you to crash an hour later.

> Golden milk: This is a blend of turmeric, ginger, natural sweetener, and unsweetened almond milk. The warm blend of milk and spices calms the stomach and can help prevent nausea and indigestion. Turmeric is a powerful source of antioxidants, which will provide your body with protection, especially when you find it hard to eat.

> (See golden milk recipe)

Dodge the dreadful nausea and morning sickness by:
- Staying hydrated. Plain water is best but can be substituted with an alternative choice listed above when needed.
- Eating lighter meals. Heavy meals can be too much for the stomach and cause nausea. Try a salad with quinoa rather than meat and potatoes

- Eating every 2 to 3 hours. I don't mean having large meals every few hours, but eating frequent small meals through the day can be much easier on your belly then three large meals. It will also keep your energy levels up!
- Have a very light breakfast as soon as you wake. Keeping some gluten-free crackers next to your bed so you can have a few first thing in the morning can keep you from getting sick. Having a little something in your belly right when you wake up may actually hold off nausea for the whole day. You may follow up with a second light breakfast such as toast or fruit later in the morning.
- Avoid spicy and over fatty foods. Eating very hot or fatty foods can cause a stomach to react. It may also give you intense heartburn. Aim for mild, simple flavours paired with lower fat dishes to ease your nausea.
- Ginger! Drinking ginger tea or chewing some dried, pure ginger whenever you are feeling nauseous is a great way to calm the stomach.
- Do NOT overeat. When you are pregnant, you may feel the urge to overeat or "eat for two" every now and then. But when you over-stuff yourself, guess what is not far behind to empty you out!

Some doctors may prescribe you an anti-nausea medication to help settle your stomach. I would highly recommend avoiding prescription drugs while pregnant, unless not taking it would be threatening to you or your baby's health.

Try to cope with morning sickness using natural remedies and only opt for the medication as your last resort. The symptoms of morning sickness should depart in the second trimester for most women, giving you the window of opportunity to cram in as many whole foods into your diet as possible. Nausea may return again in the third trimester, so do your best to fill up on the good stuff when feeling up to it.

The essentials

Aside from staying well hydrated and taking a prenatal vitamin everyday, our bodies need much more. A prenatal vitamin is just a supplement to our daily food intake to ensure we receive our recommended dosage of any nutrient we may be lacking. Although every vitamin and mineral we consume is vital to our health, there are certain nutrients that play an important role in pregnancy. In order to ensure we are getting enough of those nutrients, we need to consume a diet rich in those particular foods.

> Foliate or folic acid: For the first 4 months of pregnancy, taking a folic acid supplement or eating large amounts of foods rich in folic acid will help your baby develop normally and decrease the chance of birth defects. Foods that contain folic acid are oranges,

dark leafy greens, chickpeas, and lentils. The RDA recommends 400 mcg of foliate daily while pregnant.

Vitamin C: This is an essential nutrient for the structural protein collagen. Collagen is necessary to form and protect cartilage, skin, tendons, and bones. Foods that contain vitamin C are citrus fruits, red bell peppers, and apples. The RDA recommends 85 mg of vitamin C daily while pregnant.

Vitamin D: This is needed to maintain normal levels of phosphorus and calcium in the body, which are necessary for the development of baby's bones and teeth. Foods that contain vitamin D are fatty fish, vitamin D-fortified eggs and cereal, and fish liver oil. Direct sunshine also delivers a great amount of vitamin D, but to prevent the risk of skin cancer or for those who do not get exposure to a lot of sun, it is highly recommended that all pregnant women take a vitamin D supplement daily. The RDA recommends 200 IU's each day for pregnant women.

Vitamin A (beta-carotene and retinol): This is crucial to the development of the baby's heart, eyes, bones, lungs, and central nervous system. Vitamin A is actually split into two different types: retinol and beta-carotene. Both are found in different types of foods. Foods that contain retinol are eggs, liver, and organic cow's milk. Foods that contain beta-carotene are found in fruits and vegetables. Carrots are extremely high in this vitamin. The RDA recommends 2500 of vitamin A per day. To ensure you are getting a balance of each type of vitamin A, eat a variety of foods that contain each nutrient.

B complex: In total, there are eight different B vitamins that fall under the B complex category. They assist the body in converting food to energy and in the formation of red blood cells. The B complex is extremely important for the growth and development of the fetus. The B vitamins are found in foods such as eggs, red meat, poultry, fish, legumes, leafy greens, and nutritional yeast. Vitamin B12 can only be found in animal products. So if you consume a vegetarian or vegan diet, you must get your B12 in the form of a supplement. Because each dosage varies between the different B vitamins, eating a balanced diet of various foods or supplementing with a B complex will ensure you are getting the recommended dosage of all the B vitamins.

Calcium: This mineral is needed to help your baby to build strong bones and to maintain a healthy heart, nerves, and muscles. Ensuring you are consuming enough calcium in your diet is just as important for the mother as it is for the fetus. The lack of calcium on the mother's behalf will cause the fetus to draw calcium from the mother's bones to fulfill its own needs. This can cause the mother to become calcium deficient later in life. Foods that contain calcium are dark leafy greens, sesame seeds, canned fish with edible bones, fortified orange juice, and organic soy products. It is highly recommended for pregnant women to supplement with calcium to ensure they are reaching the recommended daily intake. The RDA recommends 1000 IU of calcium per day for pregnant women.

Iron: This is another crucial nutrient in pregnancy, since a mother's blood volume doubles during pregnancy. A higher dosage of iron is needed for the production of hemoglobin, which assists in red blood cells delivering oxygen to the body. Extra iron is especially needed in the second and third trimester for your growing baby and to prevent you from developing anemia. Foods that contain iron are red meats, legumes, vegetables, and grains. The RDA recommends 27 mg of iron per day for pregnant women

Zinc: This mineral is needed for the support of the immune system and wound healing, which comes in handy after childbirth. It is also needed for cell growth, which increases rapidly during pregnancy. Although zinc deficiencies are rare, studies shows it may be linked to miscarriages and low birth weight. Foods that contain zinc are red meats and fortified, whole-grain cereals. Shellfish also contains a good amount of zinc. The RDA recommends 11 mg of zinc per day for pregnant women.

Prevention of miscarriages

In your first trimester, the risks for a miscarriage are a lot higher than when you are in your second and third. Your fetus is starting to develop and many problems can occur, even death, if you are not extra careful. Although miscarriages are not always preventable, there are many steps you can take to ensure your baby has a healthy development.

1. Prepare your body for pre-conception: As covered in the first chapter, allowing your body to heal and re-balance by following a fertility cleanse can decrease your chances of a future miscarriage. When the body is in a healthy state, it is less likely to develop imbalances that could affect the fetus. Preparing the body with fertility cleanses will also rid the body of any toxins that could interfere with the health of a fetus. This will also help increase the circulation of blood flow in the uterus.

2. Increase the consumption of essential nutrients needed for a healthy pregnancy. Start by taking a prenatal vitamin as soon as you confirm you are pregnant. (Better yet, begin taking one prior to conception). Make sure your prenatal vitamin is a high-quality brand made from whole foods. This ensures that you are not putting any synthetic ingredients into your body. You should also be aware of what vitamins and minerals your prenatal vitamin contains. Although most prenatal vitamins do contain all of the necessary vitamins, be sure to double-check that yours contains vitamins B6, B12, and folic acid aka foliate. This combination has been shown to help prevent miscarriages due to its high levels of homocysteine.

3. Increase your amount of essential fatty acids (EFA's)! EFA's are extremely important when maintaining a healthy body. Consuming high amounts of EFA's, especially omega 3 in

your diet, is an excellent way to decrease the chances of a miscarriage. Omega 3 plays an extremely important role in fertility as it helps to reduce inflammation and aids in hormone production and balance.

4. The obvious step to reducing the chances of having a miscarriage is to reduce caffeine consumption and eliminate ALL alcohol, drugs (even prescription drugs, unless they are absolutely necessary), and cigarettes.

Necessary avoidances

Caffeine: First let's start with caffeine. Although it may be difficult to eliminate, decreasing your intake of caffeine to less than 200 mg a day will help decrease your chances of having a miscarriage. It is important to reduce or eliminate caffeine during pregnancy because it may seriously harm the growing fetus. Caffeine crosses through the placenta barrier to the fetus, and since the fetus is not fully developed, it can be hard for he or she to metabolize it. Studies have even shown caffeine can influence cell development and decrease blood flow to the placenta, which may affect the growth and development of the fetus.

Alcohol: This is one substance that every mother should refrain from completely. Some say that having small to moderate amounts of alcohol while pregnant will not harm the fetus, but do you really want to take that chance? In my personal opinion, NO amount of alcohol is safe during pregnancy. It has been proven that alcohol consumption, especially during the first 3 months of pregnancy, can have toxic effects on the fetus. Most miscarriages are caused by an abnormality in the cytoplasm of the egg that negatively affects its quality. When the quality of the egg is compromised, it automatically increases the risk of a miscarriage.

Drugs: Both drugs and prescription drugs are involved in determining the chance of a miscarriage. Although there are certain prescription medications that are necessary for some, it is important to decrease or eliminate the ones that are not. There are many side effects listed on the bottles of prescription drugs and even on some over-the-counter drugs such as the pain killer Ibuprofen, but the side effects of what these drugs can do to a fetus is unlisted and unknown. Just like the effects of alcohol on the unborn fetus, prescription drugs can act the same way and cross the placenta barrier where they can be absorbed by the fetus. Because the fetus is so delicate and undeveloped, it may not react well to the medication that it has just ingested through the mother. Although most over-the-counter and pre-scribed medications are considered safe during pregnancy, it is still best to avoid as many of these substances as possible – and especially until the 12-week period of your pregnancy has passed. Always check with your doctor before taking any new medication. Street drugs will act the same way, but are much more fatal as they are already considered dangerous when consumed by adults. Enough said: Avoid them like the plague for the health of yourself and your unborn angel.

Necessary Additives

Now that we have learned what to avoid during pregnancy, let's look at the necessary additives in the first trimester. Eating these particular foods gives you and the baby a major health advantage. These foods contain certain compounds that will benefit the both of you.

Avocado: These beautiful fruits are filled with essential fatty acids. These fatty acids are the crucial building blocks for the fetus brain and retinas. There has also been research showing essential fatty acids can prevent post-natal depression.

Purple Cabbage: This is ten times higher in vitamin C than oranges. Studies have shown that a vitamin C deficiency in newborn babies can impair mental development. This vitamin is also important for moms as it is necessary for wound healing, which will highly benefit you after childbirth.

Proteins: Proteins or amino acids, which are the building blocks of protein (and of you and your baby), are found in almost any food. They are highly over-rated and traditionally it has been thought that we need to consume a large amount of meat and dairy to meet our daily needs. Yes, proteins can be found in animal flesh, but they are also in legumes and whole grains, which are much better choices as they contain so many vitamins, minerals, and fibre. You really only need about 60 to 70 grams(.6-.7kg) of protein a day while you are pregnant – not 1 gram of protein per 1 pound of body weight, which is a little extreme. As long as you are consuming a wide variety of different foods, such as leafy greens, vegetables, whole grains, and lean animal protein, you will meet the daily requirement without any problem. The key is to consume high-quality proteins such as organic and free-range animal proteins, along with organic vegetables and whole grains when possible. This way, you lower the risk of consuming harmful antibiotics, which can cause major health effects in your baby.

Dark green vegetables: Leafy greens – such as romaine, spinach, kale, and Swiss chard – and other bulk vegetables – such as broccoli, Brussels sprouts, and asparagus – are the healthiest foods you can be eating during this trimester. They are all chock-full of calcium, vitamins A and C, foliate, and many other nutrients that are crucial to a growing baby's needs. Foliate, a much-needed nutrient during pregnancy, can reduce the risk of your baby being with born defects such as spina bifida, a developmental congenital disorder caused by the incomplete closing of the embryonic neural tube.

By taking care of your health, you are automatically taking care of your baby's health.

Chapter 4
What You Need to Know in Your Second Trimester

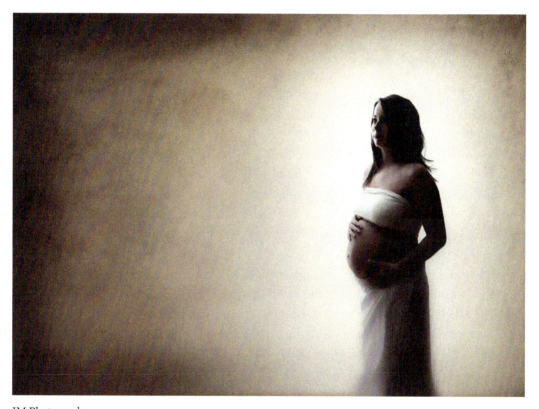

JM Photography

Now that you are in your second trimester, most of the uncomfortable symptoms that you experienced in the first trimester have probably disappeared, making this trimester "the baby boon" phase. It is also called the "honeymoon stage of pregnancy", when you can push nausea and tiredness aside and just enjoy yourself. Not every woman experiences this phase, but the ones who do, treasure it, as those pesky, past symptoms disappear and before possible new ones can appear in the third trimester.

Another great aspect of being in your second trimester is the decreased risk of having a miscarriage. When the fetus reaches the second trimester, its chances of survival go up, and your risk of miscarriage drops down to below 10 percent. The highest miscarriage rates are from 1 to 12 weeks gestation. So moms who pass this point tend to feel some reassurance.

Fetal development progresses rapidly during the second trimester. There are many great things you will uncover during this trimester, such as hearing baby's heart beat, finally being able to show off your baby bump, feeling him/her kick for the first time, and even finding out the sex of your baby!

Upping the calories

During the second trimester, your nutrient intake and caloric intake usually increases due to your growing baby. Continuing to maintain a healthy diet full of natural, whole foods, vitamins, and essential fatty acids will ensure you are still providing your unborn baby with all the nutrients he/she needs to continue developing.

Moms who are still having food aversions and morning sickness may find it hard to keep food down or even take in those healthy vegetables and fruits. If you are one of the unlucky ones who is still suffering from nausea and morning sickness and veggies just make you want to gag, continue taking your prenatal vitamin and follow the guidelines mentioned in the first trimester to help curb your nausea. Still try to do your best and consume as many whole foods as your stomach will allow.

As pregnancy becomes more of a reality, and you find yourself getting bigger, it may be more difficult to prepare healthy, home-cooked meals. The trick is to choose as many fresh foods as possible that do not require a lot of preparation work and cooking. Fresh, organic fruits and vegetables are your best bet, as you can wash and eat them the way they are. The same goes for raw nuts and seeds, which are great sources of protein and healthy fats. Having pre-boiled, organic eggs in your fridge can provide a ready-to-grab snack. Likewise, stock up your cupboards with whole-grain breads, cereals, and applesauce! Eating right, even when you're too tired to prepare food and cook, can still be simple, as long as you have a lot of low-maintenance food on hand.

Don't be scared to even ask your parents, in-laws, or better yet your partner to prepare some meals you enjoy and freeze them. On the days you don't feel like doing anything, just pop them out of the freezer, reheat, and enjoy!

During the next few months, you will also notice your body putting on more weight than before. This is completely normal, not to mention healthy. This is the time in pregnancy when many expectant women start disliking the shape of their body. Dieting at this point in your life is entirely out of the question.

Eating enough is extremely important, and restricting calories to lose weight or prevent further weight gain is detrimental to you and your baby. Remember that once your baby is born, the weight you have put on will come off within the few months following birth. A lot of moms who exercise and continue eating healthy after birth say their body looks better after having the baby than before they even became pregnant! So keep eating those calories, and once your baby is born, you can slowly start to reduce them.

In your second trimester you should be consuming about 300 extra calories a day. That's just a couple of extra servings from the different food groups. Remember that you are NOT eating for two, so I don't recommend scarfing down double of everything you make. Otherwise, your healthy weight gain will turn into an overweight pregnancy, and no one wants that.

The truth about gestational diabetes

At this point in pregnancy, you should begin to gain roughly 1-2 pounds (.4-.9kg) per week. Usually toward the end of the second trimester, a glucose-screening test will be done to test for gestational diabetes (GD). As many as one in six moms will develop this disease. GD can pose a risk to both you and your baby. GD develops when a mother's pancreas cannot produce enough insulin to help lower her blood sugar levels. GD usually disappears after a woman gives birth, but if a woman continues to have high blood sugar after birth, she has a higher chance of developing type 2 diabetes later in life.

Who is at risk for developing GD?

Those who have a greater risk of developing gestational diabetes are:

1. Women who are overweight with a BMI of 30 or over
2. Women who have had gestational diabetes in previous pregnancies
3. Women who have given birth to a previous baby that weighed over 9 pounds (4 kg)
4. Diabetes runs in your family

Prevention and management

There are ways to prevent and manage gestational diabetes. You can do so by:

1. Eating a whole-foods diet consisting of fresh fruit and vegetables, whole grains, and legumes. These foods contain high amounts of fibre, which is known to stabilize blood sugar levels and help maintain a healthy weight.

2. Staying active

3. Maintaining a healthy BMI. If you are overweight prior to becoming pregnant, do your best to bring your BMI down before you conceive.

4. Gaining the recommended weight while pregnant

What can I expect if I develop GD?

There are risks for you and baby if you do develop gestational diabetes. These risks are:

1. Giving birth to a larger baby

2. An increased need for intervention and possibly a C-section

3. An increased chance the baby will have childhood diabetes and obesity

4. An increased chance of high blood pressure and preeclampsia in the mother

5. An increased chance of the mother developing type 2 diabetes later in life

Foods to avoid

Eating a healthy, whole foods diet while living an active lifestyle is the best and easiest way to maintain a healthy pregnancy weight and reduce the risks of developing GD.

If you are at risk of developing GD, avoid the following foods:
- Processed grains: white bread, white flour, white pasta
- Sugary cereals made with refined and not whole grains
- Fried and overly fatty foods
- Candy and chocolate
- Baked goods made with refined grains, sugar, and fat
- Soda
- Sweetened fruit juices

Chapter 5
What You Need to Know in Your Third Trimester

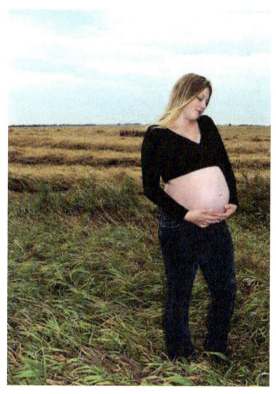

Shantel Hanson

Say good-bye to that honeymoon phase most of you moms had the chance to experience and take advantage of in your second trimester. Since this is the last trimester before you meet your little one, your old symptoms of nausea and fatigue may return and could even be worst than they were in your first trimester.

As your body requires more energy to provide for your growing baby, fatigue becomes your number one enemy. Take advantage of rest when you can, and make sure to continue eating sufficient calories to help your energy levels stay up.

In the third trimester, most moms need a to consume an additional 400 calories per day to sustain their healthy pregnancy weight. You are still aiming to gain a healthy 1-2 pounds(0.4-0.9kg) a week. Don't be alarmed that towards the end of your due date, your appetite may suddenly decrease, and you will no longer continue to gain weight. This is completely normal as your baby is finished growing, and your body is now preparing for labour and delivery.

Pesky symptoms

During the third trimester, many expectant mothers start experiencing symptoms of heart burn, constipation, gas, and fullness after even just a few bites of food. These symptoms are completely normal and are due to your baby taking up so much space inside your belly. Your uterus is now up to your ribcage, pushing all your other organs – such as your intestines and stomach – in a little bunch. This can result in more acid creeping back up the esophagus causing heartburn. Your digestive system is also working at a much slower rate. By slowing down your metabolism, your body is allowing baby to absorb as many nutrients and calories as possible.

Constipation is also very common around this time of pregnancy. If you suffer from this symptom, ramp up the amount of fibre and water in your diet to keep things moving along. You may also talk to your health practitioner about a gentle stool softener that is safe for pregnancy, if nothing else seems to be doing the trick.

If you are finding it harder to eat bigger meals or are getting too many symptoms following a meal, try consuming smaller meals every 3 hours throughout the day. This will prevent you from feeling overly stuffed and bloated and can also decrease the amount of heartburn. The good news is that this struggle of unwanted symptoms is only temporary, especially if this is your first child.

First time mothers will experience effacement, which is when your baby drops lower into the pelvic cavity. This usually happens up to a month before birth. Your poor, bunched-up organs now have some more breathing room, which decreases the chances of heartburn and shortness of breath and increases the chances of being able to consume a meal that's bigger than what you would feed a toddler. For veteran moms, effacement usually does not happen until you are in labour, unfortunately.

Pumping the iron

In your last trimester, your lack of energy could also be a sign that you're lacking in iron. Although your baby can be getting his/her recommended dosage of iron from you, low iron in pregnancy may increase the chances of preterm delivery and low birth weight. It is also associated with a higher risk of stillbirths or newborn deaths, so make sure you are getting an adequate supply of this nutrient. During your prenatal blood tests, your iron level will be checked, and if it is low, your doctor will recommend that you start taking an iron supplement.

In order to prevent an iron deficiency from arising, make sure your diet is filled with iron-rich foods such as red meat, shellfish, beans, lentils, and lots of leafy green vegetables. Avoid consuming liver during your pregnancy. It does contain high levels of iron, but it also has very high amounts of vitamin A, which can be considered dangerous and toxic to your baby. Consuming high amounts of vitamin C in your diet will also help to increase the amount of iron absorption in your body. Foods like bell peppers, citrus fruits, and green vegetables are great sources of vitamin C and should be eaten with an iron-rich food.

Developing anemia

Some women are at greater risk for developing anemia while pregnant than others. If you do suspect that you are anemic, seek the advice of a health professional immediately. You are at a greater risk for developing anemia if you:

1. Have suffered from morning sickness with lots of vomiting
2. Have had two pregnancies close together
3. Lack iron-rich foods in your diet
4. Are pregnant with more than one baby
5. Have had anemia prior to pregnancy

Symptoms

Symptoms of anemia include:

1. Feeling fatigued and weak
2. Dizziness along with shortness of breath
3. Pale skin and lips
4. Trouble focusing

The risks of developing anemia while pregnant can be very serious to you and your child. Ensure that you take precautions, especially if you suspect that you are not getting enough iron in your diet.

Risks

The risks of developing anemia are:

1. Giving birth to a preterm baby or a baby with a low birth weight
2. Having an increased chance of post-partum depression
3. Having a child who may be anemic and possibly suffer from developmental delays

Foods to include

Consuming a diet full of iron-rich foods combined with foods rich in vitamin C lowers the risk of developing anemia. Food combinations of iron and vitamin C include:

- Organic red meat and steamed broccoli
- Beans and quinoa stuffed red bell peppers
- Seafood with cooked tomatoes, kale, and peas
- Smoothie made with spinach, oranges, and berries
- Salad with dark leafy greens, chicken, and dried apricots
- Iron-fortified cereal with fresh fruit

Chapter 6
No Meat Mommies

Are you a mom who doesn't eat meat or any animal byproducts? That's no problem! Whether it is for ethical or health reasons, it is your choice to abstain from eating certain foods. However, you should be aware that your nutrition is a bit more complex than that of a meat eater and you will have to take extra caution about ensuring you are getting all the essential nutrients needed for your baby.

In some cases, vegan and vegetarians may lack certain vitamins and minerals in their diet that they are unaware of because some are only found in animal products or supplements. During pregnancy, these nutrients are extremely important in maintaining a healthy fetus. But don't worry, you don't have to give up on your specific diet and start eating a steak everyday to get what you need. You will just have to focus more on creating meals that are balanced, as well as supplementing your diet with the needed nutrients you may not be obtaining from your food.

Balance and food pairing

First things first. Balance and variety are the key components when structuring a meat-free diet. Our body must receive all the essential amino acids from protein sources to ensure a healthy functioning body. Amino acids are the building blocks of protein. They are responsible for proper brain function, immune system maintenance, bone and tissue maintenance, and even the quality of sleep. Many vegan and vegetarian diets lack in amino acids, including an array of important B vitamins. In order to ensure your body is receiving all the essential amino acids, you will need to properly balance meals.

When preparing your meal, be sure to include a serving of grains and a serving of legumes together. By doing so, you are creating a meal that contains all the essential amino acids, minus the meat! Here are just a few of my favourite whole grains and legumes:

Whole Grains (not all are gluten-free, but all are unprocessed)
- Amaranth
- Barley
- Buckwheat
- Bugler
- Millet
- Oats
- Unrefined wheat
- Quinoa
- Brown or wild rice
- Spelt
- Rye
- Sprouted grains
- Legumes
- Adzuki beans
- Black beans
- Black-eyed peas
- Chick peas
- Edamame
- Fava beans
- Lima beans
- Red and white kidney beans
- Navy beans
- Lentils

By pairing these two food groups together, you are also providing your body with a good balance of complex carbs and lean protein, as well as with sustained energy and plenty of fibre.

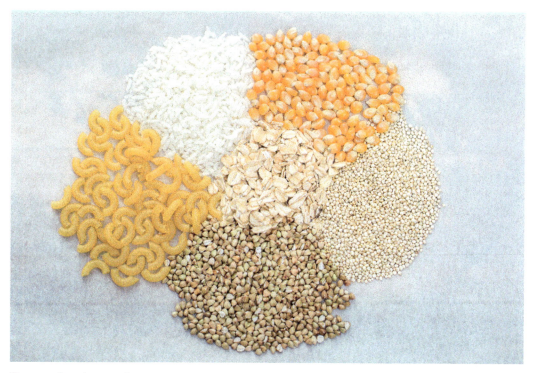

You come first photography

It's all about the fat

The second most important additive to balance a meal is fat! Not just any fat, but the healthy, brain food kind – the essential fatty acids (EFA's), omega 3, polyunsaturated and monounsaturated. These fats are necessary for maintaining good health and for the growing fetus. They are essential for the protection of your brain and other organs and also help you stay full and satisfied after a meal. Essential fatty acids not only benefit you internally, they also benefit you externally by providing your skin with the lubrication it needs to stay silky and smooth. Adding just a small amount of fat with every meal will give you the recommended amount.

Fat deficiencies

Fat deficiency can cause serious consequences and can eventually lead to depression, dietary energy defiance, and worse, malnutrition. ADHD and low IQ's are also associated with essential fatty acid deficiency. Not consuming adequate amounts of EFA's while pregnant can increase the risk of preeclampsia, high blood pressure, and premature birth. EFA's are crucial for optimal development of the fetal nervous system.

Although there are numerous symptoms of EFA deficiency, here are the top 5:

1. Low mental energy
2. Dry hair and skin, and brittle nails
3. Poor concentration
4. Constipation
5. Irritability

Supplementing your diet with a fish oil (for vegetarians who consume fish) or a plant-based fatty acid blend is recommended throughout pregnancy to aid in the prevention of an EFA deficiency.

Fat-soluble vitamins

Fat also plays an important role in the absorption of certain vitamins. Fat-soluble vitamins such as A, D, E, and K, can only be broken down when there is fat present. Eating a meal that consists of chickpeas, rice, and broccoli will not give you the same benefit compared to if it were a meal consisting of chickpeas, rice, broccoli, and avocado.

Here are some essential fatty acids to add to every meal. Add only moderate amounts as fats are very high in calories and can be easily over-consumed:
- Avocado
- Extra virgin coconut and olive oil
- Flax seeds (ground or oil)
- Any type of nut or seed
- Hemp hearts
- Coconut meat
- Free-range eggs
- Chia seeds

Vitamins and minerals

The last component to preparing a healthy and balanced meat-free meal is the vitamins and minerals! Although you do get a good dose of certain vitamins and minerals from your grains and legumes, the load of it all comes from fruits and vegetables. Fruits and vegetables are chock-full of nutrients; much more so than grains, starches, and legumes. They also contain plenty of fibre and antioxidants. You should be aiming to consume about seven 1/2 cup servings of non-starchy vegetables and four 1/2 cup servings of fruit per day.

Because there is such an enormous list of vegetables and fruit, I have listed the ones that contain the most nutrients and that are considered super foods for the body.

Fruits:
- Apples: Contain antioxidants called flavonoids, which are great for reducing the chance of developing diabetes and asthma
- Bananas: Loaded with potassium, which can help lower high blood pressure
- Blackberries: A powerful antioxidant that may help reduce the risk of stroke and cancer
- Blueberries: Number one antioxidant; they can lower the risk of developing Parkinson's and Alzheimer's
- Cantaloupe: High in the antioxidant beta-carotene, which may help reduce the risk of developing cataracts
- Cherries: An excellent antioxidant that can help relieve arthritis and gout
- Cranberries: These antibacterial fruits can help treat and prevent urinary tract infections.
- Figs: High in fibre, may reduce the risk of heart disease
- Goji berries: Nutrient powerhouse, containing six vitamins, 21 minerals, and a load of antioxidants
- Oranges: Oranges are a good source of foliates, an important vitamin for pregnant women that can help prevent neural tube defects in their infants.
- Grapes: Grapes contain the antioxidant resveratrol that may help prevent heart disease
- Pomegranate: Pomegranates contain antioxidant tannins, which may protect the heart.
- Papaya: Contain papain, an enzyme that aids digestion. They are also extremely high in vitamin A, which aids in maintaining healthy skin.
- Raspberries: Raspberries are rich in ellagic acid, an antioxidant that may help prevent cervical cancer.
- Watermelon: Over 92 percent water, watermelon is a great way to stay hydrated, especially when that dreadful morning sickness kicks in.

And of course the veggies:
- Asparagus: Loaded with fibre, foliate, vitamins A, C, E, and K, and antioxidants
- Broccoli: Contains high amounts of calcium, magnesium and potassium, which can help maintain a healthy nervous system, blood pressure and bone health.
- Beets: Beets are shown to provide antioxidant, anti-inflammatory, and detoxification support.
- Bell peppers: These are a good source of vitamin C and also contain high amounts of fibre. They are also an antioxidant. High in potassium, this vegetable helps keep your fluids and minerals balanced in your body, enhances muscle function, and regulates blood pressure.
- Carrots: These "good for the eyes" orange vegetables contain high amounts of vitamin A (beta-carotene), which is essential for healthy vision. It can also help slow down the aging process!

- Kale: This green veggie has more iron than beef! Iron is essential for good health, as it transports oxygen to various parts of the body and aids in cell growth, proper liver function, and more.
- Spinach: One cup of spinach has nearly 20% of the RDA of dietary fibre, which aids in digestion, prevents constipation, maintains low blood sugar, and curbs overeating.
- Onions: Onions contain phytochemicals that support the working of vitamin C in the body, improving your body's immune system. They also contain high amounts of chromium, which is essential for the regulation of blood sugar.
- Summer squash (also known as yellow squash): This vegetable is very high in vitamin c and potassium. It also contains antioxidants to keep free radicals at bay, decreasing the risk of developing cancer.
- Tomatoes: Are a good source of citamins A, C, K, foliate, and potassium. Tomatoes also contain a high level of the nutrient lycopene, which is an antioxidant compound that gives tomatoes their red colour. There have also been studies showing that this nutrient can prevent and treat cancer. Lycopene levels in tomatoes actually increase when cooked!

Aside from consuming all of these wonderful foods to provide you with a nutrient-dense, vegetarian diet, additional supplements are still very important. There are some vitamins you cannot obtain enough of just from consuming foods alone, and that group of vitamins is called B vitamins or the B complex. B vitamins are a group of water-soluble vitamins that play important roles in cell metabolism. The B complex also includes one of the most vital nutrients needed for a healthy pregnancy – folic acid.

Since most B vitamins are primarily found in animal foods – although high amounts are shown to be stored in nutritional yeast, taking an additional B vitamin complex will ensure you are getting enough of this wonderful vitamin. B vitamins are usually included in your daily multi or prenatal vitamin, but an additional source is recommended if following a strict, no meat diet plan.

With this being said, you now have every nutrient you need to complete a balanced meal. So continue to enjoy your animal-product-free lifestyle and don't worry about lacking certain vitamins for yourself and your baby.

Chapter 7
Mind and Body Detox

Environmental toxins

I often get asked questions from my expecting clients, not just about certain foods that may contain toxic ingredients, but also about certain household items that may be considered toxic – if not necessarily to us, to an unborn child.

We are exposed to a world where pollution is increasing, and more and more products are being produced to make our life easier. We now have things like cleaning supplies, laundry detergent, lotions, shampoo, plastic water bottles, and even pregnancy products like stretchmark cream and oils.

As unfortunate as it is, many of the products on today's shelves contain poisonous toxins that can be a hazard to you and your baby. While you can't avoid cleaning your house, your clothes, or yourself because of the fear that toxins in your products may be negatively affecting your health, you can find natural alternatives and know what to avoid when seeking out new products.

What to avoid

Here is a list of some of the deadliest household products. You should do your best to avoid these and find alternatives to replace them right away.

- Air fresheners: The secret behind air fresheners and their magic to make any odour disappear is that they actually interfere with your ability to smell. They do this by releasing nerve-deadening agents into the air, which you breath in accompanied with the harsh smell of chemical scents.
- Windex or other multi-surface cleaners that contain ammonia: Ammonia is a very volatile chemical that is very damaging to your eyes, respiratory tract, and skin.

- Bleach: This chemical is a strong corrosive, which can irritate or burn the skin, eyes, and even the respiratory tract. It can also cause vomiting or coma if ingested. Never mix ammonia or bleach together as it can form and release deadly fumes.
- Dishwasher detergents: Most of these products contain the chemical chlorine, which is highly concentrated in a dry form. This is the number one cause of child poisonings according to the poison control centre.
- Laundry detergent: Most detergents contain the following chemicals: Sodium lauryl sulfate (SLS)/sodium laureth sulfate (SLES) 1, and 4-dioxane NPE (nonylphenol ethoxylate) phosphates. These chemicals are not only hazardous to your health; they are also harmful to the environment.
- Hair dye: Although not a household cleaning product, hair dye is commonly used by women even during pregnancy. As there is still some controversy about expectant mothers using hair dye, try to avoid dying your hair in the first trimester or sticking to highlights rather than full colour as the chemicals don't saturate the scalp. However, hair dye is packed full of heavy metals, which can be absorbed by the scalp and into the bloodstream. Letting your roots grow in for 9 whole months may not be the most pleasant thing in the world, but you are avoiding the risk of those colouring agents affecting your baby.

There are many hair dyes made from henna, which do not contain harsh chemicals. These are much safer to use while pregnant. Henna is all natural and made from the dried leaves of the plant called lawsonia. Most henna dyes contain red hues, but there are also brands that are formulated for brunettes and those with black hair.

You may not get the salon quality, but you can definitely get the satisfaction that you are protecting your fetus. Most commercial hair dyes contain two toxic chemicals called phenylenediamine and tar coal. Studies have shown that repeated exposure to these chemicals increases the risk of certain cancers in humans. Tar coal can also contain the heavy metals and arsenic and lead, which are shown to disrupt our body's hormones and can also contribute to causing cancer.

Not only is hair dye a concern with expectant mothers, there are also many products that are applied directly onto our skin that contain these deadly toxins, and yet they are passed as being safe for human use! Most shampoos, conditioners, body washes, face lotions, nail polishes, deodorants, and even lip balms contain harmful chemicals that your skin absorbs and that can easily cross the placenta barrier into the bloodstream where it is absorbed by your baby.

What's wrong with these toxins?

In addition to causing minor problems, such as skin irritations and digestive issues, these toxins are suspected of contributing to much more serious health issues, such as multiple sclerosis, heart disease, cancer, and Alzheimer's. To avoid these toxic chemicals from being absorbed into your bloodstream, avoid products that have these chemicals listed in their ingredients:

- Diethanolamine (DEA)
- Propylene glycol
- Sodium lauryl sulfate
- Parabens, phthalates, polyethylene glycol, aluminum

Here's a tip for moms-to-be: Not all your pregnancy lotions and oils, and even your recently purchased baby products, are considered safe, so be sure to double-check those products for these sneaky chemicals. Most products that are commonly used to prevent and treat stretchmarks contain petroleum as a main ingredient. Studies show petroleum is considered a carcinogenic – aka cancerous! Your best bet for avoiding these toxic chemicals is to search for an all-natural alternative or better yet, make what you can from scratch. Raw coconut oil acts as a perfect alternative to any store-bought stretchmark cream. Coconut oil contains high amounts of vitamin E, which is essential for healthy skin.

D.I.Y.M: Do it yourself mamas!

Many moms today are saving money and their health by making homemade products for cleaning and hygiene. Not only is it saving them a pretty penny, it is also contributing to a less polluted environment. It may sound complicated, but making your own household products couldn't be more simple. With just a few ingredients, you can make anything from dish soaps, shampoo, glass cleaner, to even body lotions and lip balm – not to mention baby products. Here are some homemade recipes for family hygiene and household items:

All-purpose cleaning spray

    1 part vinegar
    1 part water
    .5 part lemon or lime juice
    Drops of your favourite essential oil (lavender, tea tree oil, etc.)
    Combine all ingredients in a spray bottle and shake well.
    Spray on surfaces and wipe clean with a cloth

Mirror cleaner

1 part white vinegar
1 part 70% rubbing alcohol
1 part pure or distilled water
Combine all ingredients in a spray bottle and shake well. Spray on mirrors and wipe clean with a microfibre cloth or newspaper for a streak-free shine!

Organic homemade lotion

1/4 cup coconut oil
1/2 cup of almond or olive oil (can infuse with herbs first if desired)
1/4 cup beeswax
Optional: 1 teaspoon vitamin E oil
Optional: 2 tablespoons shea butter or cocoa butter
Vanilla essential oil
Combine ingredients in a 16 oz mason jar. Fill a saucepan with a couple of inches of water and place over medium heat. Place the jar in the pan with the water. The mixture will melt as the water heats. Stir occasionally. When all ingredients are completely melted, pour into a glass jar with a lid. Mason jars work great.

"No poo" shampoo

Rinse your hair with 1 tbsp of baking soda then rinse with 1 tbsp of cider vinegar for an amazing hair wash that doesn't strip your hair of its natural oils. Try rubbing a few drops of orange or rose essential oil into your damp, washed hair for a delicious, fresh scent!

Epsom salt bath soak

1 cup of Epsom salts
1/2 cup dried flower petals
1 tbsp of extra virgin olive oil
5-10 drops of lavender essential oil
Run a hot bath and fill with the Epsom salt mixture. Soak and enjoy.

Organic baby oil

1/2 cup olive oil
1/2 cup almond oil
5-10 drops of candeluna and chamomile oil
1 capsule of vitamin E (cut the tip off and drain oil into mixture)
Combine all ingredients in a glass mason jar. Massage a penny size amount of oil on baby's body after bath.

Baby bum powder

1 cup of arrow root powder
Tbsp of ground chamomile and lavender leaves
Combine ingredients in a small glass mason jar and mix well. Using a cotton ball, pat a small amount on baby's bottom after diaper changes.

Herbal healing baby wipes

1 to 2 cups of pure spring water
1/4 cup of aloe vera gel
2 to 3 drops of tea tree oil

2 to 3 drops of lavender oil

Tbsp candeluna oil

Combine all ingredients together in a small bowl and set aside. Lay layers of baby wash cloths or cut-up squares of fabric or paper towels inside an empty baby wipe container. Pour liquid blend on top and saturate wipes completely. Use during diaper changes.

Stress mess

We have now detoxified your body of chemical-ridden foods and toxic household products. Just by making these small changes to your lifestyle, you have provided your baby with a safe and healthy environment for him/her to grow and strive in until he/she is ready to make their way into the world.

Towards the end of your pregnancy, many unpleasant stressors may arise which can begin to negatively affect you, physically and mentally. It is important to deal with these stressors before you go into labour as it will make your birth experience more pleasant and decrease the chance that your baby will be born stressed.

Much of the stress you will experience in this stage comes from factors such as weight gain, lack of sleep, excitement and anxiety for the "big day", body pain and aches, and the big one, hormonal changes. Once you learn to relax and conquer these stressors, you will go into labour with more strength and confidence, and most importantly, calmness.

Coping mechanisms

The following are some great ways of coping with unwanted stressors:

Meditation: Meditation is an excellent way to relax emotionally and physically. By practising breathing and extending your spine, you are removing a great amount of pressure from your back and other joints. This can bring you some relief and allow you to feel more comfortable for the remainder of your pregnancy.

Find a dark, quiet room where you won't be interrupted. Sit upon a soft pillow with your legs crossed and your hands placed palms up on top of your knees. Taking deep breaths in and out, clear your mind and body of any negative energy. Practise meditation twice a day, 10 minutes in the morning and 10 minutes before bed for maximum effect. This is also a great way to calm and relieve your partner of any stress he is experiencing at this moment as well.

Prenatal yoga: Prenatal yoga is one of the best practices you can do for yourselfyou're your baby. Although prenatal yoga can be done from the start of your pregnancy, many women benefit from it more towards the end. There are numerous ways that practising yoga can bring you to peace with yourself during this stressful time.

1. Brings balance. During pregnancy, as your belly begins to grow and grow, the weight of the baby is shifted towards you. This can cause you to feel wobbly and unbalanced. Our hormones are also unbalanced at this time due to the increase in estrogen and progesterone. While practising yoga, you focus deeply on the poses and your breathing, and this can help rebalance you physically and emotionally.

2. Increases circulation. Increasing circulation is very important during pregnancy, as expectant mothers tend to have a decrease in circulation as their pregnancy progresses. This can leave you with swelling and those unfortunate leg cramps. Yoga can dramatically increase blood circulation during practice and help reduce swelling. Increased circulation is also beneficial to the baby.

3. Increases strength and flexibility. These two physical factors decrease during pregnancy due to a reduction in physical activity and mobility. Gaining strength within your body is essential for bone and joint health. With gentle yoga poses, you are able to allow your joints to relax and muscles to become strong. This will help eliminate aches and pains – and especially back pain.

4. Helps you to be calm: Prenatal yoga is another wonderful way on top of meditation that can help you relax. Deep breathing and focus brings your mind and body into a relaxed state, which can lead to more optimal sleep patterns and better digestion!

5. Connects you with your baby: Is there a more perfect way to bond with the baby inside the womb than with a little yoga? During practice, all your thoughts are focused and you are present in the moment. Feel your belly as the energy is transferred from you to your fetus and vice versa. Being zoned into your inner spirit and becoming more aware of what's within you will allow you to connect with your child on a spiritual level. It's amazing how much more we can feel when we are focused. Baby's movements become so surreal, we can almost envision what he or she is doing in there.

6. Prepares you for labour: This is the big one! As the big event gets closer and closer, yoga helps prepare the body and the mind by increasing focus, strength, and confidence. Breathing techniques during practice will benefit you during labour as well as joint stabilizing poses will allow for an easier childbirth. Yoga will also benefit you on a cardiovascular level and prepare you for the tiring, long labour you might endure.

Oat milk bath: Why not skip the traditional bubble bath and opt for a more relaxing oat milk bath. Start by filling a small piece of cheesecloth with 2 tbsp of rolled oats, 1 tbsp of whole milk powder, 2 tsp. of olive oil, 1 tbsp of dried flower petals, and a few drops of your favourite essential oil. (Lavender works wonders before bed). Fold up all the ends of the cheesecloth to form a little sack and tie the top with elastic. In a bath full of warm water, soak the sack in the water and gently massage your skin. The gentle fragrances will leave you relaxed while the oat, oil, and milk blend will soften your skin.

Journalling: I highly recommend journalling to my clients, and not only with food, but also with thoughts. During periods of high stress, channel those stressors onto the paper by expressing what you are feeling during that moment. By doing so, the stress goes into the ink and onto the paper, rather than being bottled up inside you. You can also journal the good things that are happening to you during pregnancy. You then can look back after your child has been born and revisit all those wonderful experiences. Nothing is more beautiful then being able to share those memories with your child after he or she is grown up.

Not only have you made hard sacrifices in ignoring your cravings for artificially coloured Cheetos and your morning coffee, you have made your body into a sacred temple for your little angel. Feel proud and successful. I'm sure some of this was a challenge, but you did it, and all the complications you have avoided are because you were strong. You are what is defined as a caring and loving mother, putting your child first.

But what happens after all of this begins to come to an end in your last few weeks of pregnancy? What was all the mood swings and having to avoid colouring your hair for 9 months worth? Where do you go from here as you've prepared your body for conception and for pregnancy?

Well, mommies-to-be, you are now about to begin the preparation for your baby's birth. This will probably be the most exciting stage since you found out that you were pregnant. In just a few weeks, all the challenges and rollercoasters you have gone through – mentally, physically, and emotionally – will be completely worth it as you welcome your new member of the family into this beautiful world.

Chapter 8
35 Weeks and Up

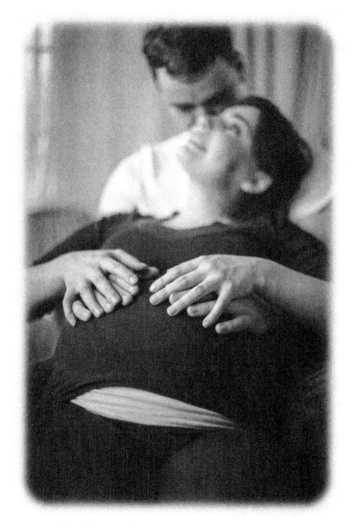

You come first photography

Well you've made it. You are still alive and thriving. Sure, mostly everything you smell and eat makes you sick; your ankles and fingers look like someone just injected you full of sodium water; you have aches and pains everywhere in your body; and your mood changes more times in a day then your television channels. But, hey, you are finally here, the last stage of pregnancy before you meet your little sweet pea.

I'm sure things are running through your mind and those 10-minute Google searches and birth videos are making you think, "What did I just get my self into? How do I prepare my body, mind, and soul for this exciting yet painful experience that I am about to embark on?" The answer is easy: Preparation. It all begins here.

Whether or not you are seeing a midwife or a doctor for all of your prenatal check-ups, you probably have been provided with some information about what to expect in the labour and delivery. If not, that's okay. I'm here to guide you on all the techniques of natural childbirth and how you can prepare your body ahead of time for the most exciting moment of your life.

Birth prep

Having a natural childbirth requires patience, strength, technique, and most of all, willpower. Sometimes it can be easier said than done. We will begin by focusing on supplements and preparations that can be taken to help ease labour, induce labour if you are overdue, prevent unnecessary interventions, and recover after birth. If you are currently seeing a midwife, she will mostly be on your side for doing everything possible to ensure a natural birth experience. However, some doctors might not agree, as their main priority is delivering a healthy baby in a short amount of time. So it is best to be prepared and know exactly what you are in for.

At 35 weeks, with only 5 weeks to go, you have a perfect window of opportunity to begin birth preparation. You may also wish to write up a birth plan to give to your doctor or midwife. A birth plan is an excellent tool for mothers who have a good idea of exactly what they want when they give birth. Although some birth plans may not go 100 percent as planned because of necessary interventions and complications that can arise during labour, it's still an excellent tool to provide a guideline of how you want things to go when you get to the hospital or birthing centre. Your doctor or midwife, as well as the labour and delivery nurses, should be given a copy of your plan as soon as you're admitted to the hospital. You can even give your delivery doctor a copy prior to your due date, so that he or she is aware ahead of time, if you have already been assigned an L&D doctor at this time.

Birth plans should include things like:
- If you chose to have a natural birth and/or what types of pain medications you prefer
- What positions you would like to try in the labour and birthing stage

- If you prefer to have certain pain alternatives present such as music or a birth pool
- Who you would like to be present in the delivery room with you
- What not to offer you or the baby as some doctors and nurses will automatically assume you want or need pain medications and will keep asking you. It is best to have it written down if you definitely do not wish to receive any pain medication. Also, for your newborn baby, most doctors assume that you want your child vaccinated on the day of birth, whereas some mothers do not wish to inject these substances into a living creature hours after being born. List any substances that you do not wish you or your baby to receive in your birth plan!

Birth plans may also contain information for your baby after birth, such as if you want to be roomed with your baby 24-7 after delivery, if you wish to have the baby latch on for immediate breastfeeding after delivery, if you plan on cord blood banking, and/or any other post-delivery requests you have.

Your birth plan does not have to be long, nor does it have to be super detailed. You can write one up yourself from scratch or you can simply download a template, which are usually available on any pregnancy website. Whichever way you chose to go, a birth plan may come in handy and prevent all kinds of annoying questions you will most likely get asked in labour and delivery. For moms wanting to have a natural birth with no interventions, this is a highly recommended tool to have.

Bring the bag

Mamas! Don't forget your hospital bag! This should be packed and ready to go in a convenient place by 36 weeks. You can easily find lists online that tell you exactly what to bring and what not to bring, and if you still aren't sure, ask your hospital or doctor. Some hospitals carry the majority of necessities for you and your baby, but in some provinces and/or states, they require you to bring most of the essentials yourself. It's always good to double-check and be prepared just in case.

Unfortunately, your hospital is most likely not to carry any natural, organic hygiene products for you and baby, so bringing your own from home may ease your mind. I've provided a list of natural products and other helpful items that you can pack with you in your hospital bag.

1. Comfy, loose-fitting clothes made from organic cotton such as baggy t-shirts or night gowns, yoga pants, thick socks or slippers, nursing bras, granny panties (as I don't think you want to ruin your best pair of bloomers!), and a light house coat.
2. Gadgets such as an iPod if you wish to have music playing. Consider creating a play list with a mixture of both soothing and relaxing music as well as more upbeat music in case you

need a boost of motivation here and there. Cellphones, cameras, video recorders, and of course their chargers are also great items to bring to capture the moment.

3. Natural hygiene products such as shampoo and conditioner, body wash for you and baby, non-petroleum-based diaper ointment, lotion, organic sanitary pads, deodorant, toothpaste and mouth wash, arnica cream (reduces pain and inflammation), essential oils, and a stool softener.

4. Food and beverages. This one may be a hit or miss depending on how you are feeling during labour and if it is safe for you to eat. In some cases, if a mother ends up having to be induced or a C-section needs be performed, most doctors advise you not to eat as it can cause complications in the procedure. So if you know this will be happening to you, make sure you fill up on a nutritious meal beforehand.

If not, it's great to bring light and easy-to-eat snacks with you. Not that you'll have an insane appetite when you are in pain, but snacks can provide you with little boosts of energy to help you pull through. Items like dates, trail mix, fruit or fruit bars, and veggies and dip are great snacks that are loaded with fibre and nutrients. Don't forget the coconut water, which is filled with potassium and electrolytes, perfect for keeping you hydrated and feeling refreshed.

Natural induction

Now that you are moving further along in your pregnancy and have almost reached full term (which most health care professionals consider to be 37 weeks), 35 weeks is a safe zone to begin taking any supplements and taking part in birth preparation exercises. However, you should have the okay from your doctor or midwife as some of these suggestions and strategies are not recommended if you are considered a high-risk pregnancy.

You've probably heard many old wives tales and even midwives talking about the different ways to prepare and naturally induce your body for labour when the time is right. While some of these "tricks" are just stories, there have actually been some proven methods to help ease labour and birth.

Red raspberry leaf tea: The red raspberry leaf is a pale-green leaf produced by the raspberry plant. It has been used for many years by pregnant women to help tone their uterus and aid in the preparation of childbirth. It is also suggested that drinking red raspberry leaf tea may shorten labour with no side effects. It is recommended that women begin drinking this tea (also available in capsule form if you cannot stomach the tea) at 28 to 34 weeks and continue to term. Some midwives may even suggest drinking one cup a day from pre-conception to term. This tea is also filled with plenty of nutrients like vitamin C and also contains antioxidants. Here are the recommended dosages:

- Tea:
  - ✓ Second trimester: 2 cups a day
  - ✓ Third trimester: 4 to 5 cups a day
- Capsules: 2, 400 mg capsules, 3 times daily with meals from 32 weeks to term

Evening primrose oil (EPO): EPO is believed to contain prostaglandins, similar to the ones contained in sperm, that can help to ripen the cervix and may prevent you from going past your due date. Although there isn't too much evidence backing this supplement for labour and birth, many midwives swear by it and it is considered a safe supplement during the end of your pregnancy. EPO is also an essential fatty acid, so if it doesn't work for labour, it will at least provide your body with many other health benefits. Here are the recommended dosages:

- ✓ 500 to 1000 mg, 2x daily from 36-38 weeks, although it is considered safe to begin orally at 34 weeks.
- ✓ 500 to 1000 mg, 3x daily from 38-40 weeks. Another suggestion that may be more effective is to continue taking the oral dosage of 1000 mg, then clip off the end of 1 or 2 capsules (2000 mg) and insert them vaginally, close to the cervix. Be sure to do this at nighttime before bed and use a panty liner, as it is a messy process.

There are other supplements to induce labour, such as caster oil and blue and black cohosh, but these are a lot more harsh to the body and should only be issued if the labour process is too slow or if you are overdue. There are also plenty of other non-supplemental procedures to try on their own or in addition to supplements. So go ahead and have fun. Just remember that no matter what you do, your baby will not come before he/she is ready. So these little tricks may not speed up labour unless your body is ready to do so. But, it's worth a try!

S.E.X: Yep, that's right. A little or a lot of intimate, or not-so-intimate love making can help with speeding up labour and getting things on a role. Studies have shown that sperm contains prostaglandins that can help soften the cervix. Softening the cervix allows the baby's head to become more engaged, which puts more pressure on the cervix for the water to break or to start bringing on the contractions. No protection is needed this time! Another great advantage about having sex is that orgasms can also bring on contractions by causing the uterus to contract. So ladies, the more you can have, the better your chances of bringing on labour.

Nipple stimulation: This is another great technique for women to try themselves or to have their partner do. Stimulating the nipples has been known to stimulate the uterus into contracting. Touching, tweaking, or lightly twisting and pinching each nipple for about 15 minutes once or twice a day can help bring on contractions. Although some women have reported this trick does help their uterus to contract, it also stops as soon as the nipple stimulation stops. Others have done one session of nipple stimulation and have gone into labour! It all depends on your body and if your baby is ready to make his/her way out. Nipple stimulation can also be done by using a breast pump. Just watch out for any milk production as we want to save that colostrum (the yellowish liquid your breasts first produce prior to milk) for baby.

Walking: The simplest way to help your labour progress is walking. Walking during pregnancy helps the baby efface (drop down into the pelvis) due to the gravitational pull. This puts pressure on your cervix and may help prime it for labour. It can also help labour progress to the point where you are feeling steady contractions. If walking isn't doing the trick, try climbing up and down the stairs for a little more of a challenge. And if all else fails, at least you've done your body good and given it a workout!

Mmmm… spicy: Some people believe that eating spicy food can actually bring on labour. The spicy food can irritate your intestines and that can cause your uterus to contract. Although there is no proven evidence that eating spicy foods induces labour, it's worth the shot and may help relieve some of that pesky constipation.

Acupuncture: The practice of acupuncture is done by inserting needles into certain pressure points on the body. This technique can stimulate uterine activity and get labour into action. Many experts and moms swear this technique is a natural and successful way to induce labour.

Acupressure: This is quite similar to acupuncture, but rather than poking the body's pressure points with needles, acupressure involves putting pressure on specific points on your body with just your fingertips to stimulate uterine activity. The two main pressure points that can be used to induce labour are the webbing between your thumb and index finger and the inside of your leg about four finger widths above the ankle bone.

Bouncing on a ball: Using a birthing ball to bounce on may seem like a ton of fun, but it can also be very useful in helping the baby drop down in to the pelvis and eventually stimulating labour to begin. Even rolling your hips side to side can do the trick and also help relieve some of that horrible back pain.

Perennial massage: Although doing perennial massages will not induce or speed up labour, it may prevent tearing that can sometimes occur when a baby is being pushed out through the vagina. A tear can be quite small or at other times very large where stiches are required. Perennial massages may also decrease the chance of having an episiotomy, in which the skin between the vagina and anus is cut to prevent tearing. Having a tear or episiotomy can be very painful, and even more painful during recovery, so doing daily perineum massages can help pre-stretch and lubricate this area to prevent tearing.

Start off by making sure your hands or your partner's hands, as he can do this for you too, are clean and sanitized. Pre-soaking in a warm bath may help soften things up so that it is easier to perform this massage. Lean back in a comfortable position (a bed with pillows behind your head works well), and lubricate your fingers and perineum with a water-based lubricant, or even better, a natural vegetable oil. (Some women even use evening primrose oil because of its cervical softening properties).

Place your or your partner's thumbs about 1 to 1.5 inches inside your vagina. Press downward and to the sides at the same time. Gently and firmly keep stretching until you feel a slight burning, tingling, or stinging sensation. This procedure should not be painful. With your thumbs, hold the pressure steady for about two minutes or until the area becomes a little numb and you can really feel the stretch.

As you keep pressing with your thumbs, slowly and gently massage back and forth over the lower half of your vagina, working the lubricant or oil into the tissues. Continue doing this for about 3-4 minutes. As you massage, pull outward on the lower part of the vagina with your thumbs hooked inside. Stretching the skin this way imitates the stretching that will occur when baby's head passes through the vagina, lessening the chance of a tear. Do this massage once or twice per day, starting around the 34th week of pregnancy up until you have started labour. This gives you plenty of time to stretch yourself out before it is baby's turn.

Even though not all of these techniques have been proven successful in inducing or speeding up labour, they are all natural and have no harmful side effects if you are having a healthy pregnancy thus far. But remember, if your baby is not ready to come, these processes won't be beneficial, so don't be too disappointed. Your little one will be coming soon enough.

Birthing techniques

Another great way to prepare your body for labour and birth is by attending a birthing class. Many classes focus on natural births and techniques such as the Bradley method or hypnobirthing. These classes will help prepare your body for what it is about to go through. Relaxation and breathing techniques are the common discussions that are had during these birthing classes. Some of these different techniques work for some, but not for others. I believe the best way is to find what works for you, whether or not you were told you should do something specific. If it's not working, find something else. Only you will know what comforts you and what will get you through giving birth. Some women think they are completely prepared and know prior to labour exactly what techniques they will be using, but once labour pain strikes, their plans and techniques go out the window. This is where your body takes over and tells you what to do; all you have to do is listen.

If you aren't interested in taking a birthing class and would rather listen to your own inner voice or do your own research, here are some handy relaxation tips that can give you a good idea on what to try or focus on when labour begins.

Breathing: Slow, deep breathing is best used during the early stages of labour, when pain is not the most intense. Slow, deep breaths may help relax the body and help manage the pain of contractions. Take a slow, deep breath through the nose and out the mouth. Repeat whenever a contraction begins and continue through until the contraction is over. Slow breathing techniques are best done when combined with other relaxation techniques such as visualization or meditation.

As labour begins to progress, and more intensely painful contractions begin, shallow, more accelerated breaths are best used. This begins with a deep breath, followed by faster and shallower breaths when contractions are occurring. By focusing on breathing, the mother make take her mind away from the pain and concentrate more on her breathing techniques. Accelerated breathing is also effective when used to control the urge to push before the baby is ready to be delivered.

During the final stage of labour, when mom is getting ready to push, she may start to feel intense pain and panic as she worries about delivering naturally with no pain medication. According to the American pregnancy Association, variable breathing can be of great benefit. This type of breathing consists of deep, long breaths, followed by accelerated, light breaths in between. Alternating intense, quick breaths with long, deep breaths can help the mother focus less on the contractions and more on her breathing. The pattern of "Hee-Hee-Hoo" breathing is what many women believe is the most beneficial in helping to deal with pain during this stage of labour.

Hypnobirthing: Hypnobirthing is a unique, relaxed, natural childbirth, enhanced by hypnosis techniques. This method is usually taught in classes where you will learn the different techniques of deep relaxation, visualization, and self-hypnosis. Hypnobirthing is specially designed for natural births to help mothers achieve a more comfortable labour and birth. It strongly encourages a natural, calm, and peaceful pregnancy and birth. Rather than teaching you how to cope with the pain, hypnobirths focus more on the premise that childbirth does not have to be painful as long as the mother is relaxed and properly prepared.

Music and lighting: Setting a peaceful and cozy environment for birth is what some mothers swear by to get them through this miraculous experience. Because some mothers aren't fortunate enough or do not wish to have an at-home birth, most hospitals and birth centres allow for some modifications such as dimmed lighting and soft music to help mom feel more at home. Although having lit candles is permitted in this situation, unless you are planning to deliver in your own home, flameless candles can be purchased and set up among the delivery room for an even more relaxing environment.

Sounds play just as much of an important role as the visual aspects. Some women wish to have soft or gentle music playing in the background to help them focus on relaxation while they are in labour. There is also the option of sound effects rather than music, such as crickets or ocean waves that may be just as relaxing or even more relaxing during labour. So why not bring your iPod and sound machine and experiment with different noises. If nothing works for you and you would rather have silence, turn it off. It is better to have more options to choose from than none at all. So bring a music player, and if you choose not to use it, don't.

Pictures: Some mothers find it comforting to bring a picture into the delivery room to keep them motivated and inspired. First-time moms may bring a picture of their baby's ultrasound to help remind them that all this pain and uncomfortable labour is completely worth it! For mothers who already have children, bringing a family picture may also bring the motivation that soon there will be another addition to the family. Others may prefer to bring a picture of a specific scene that inspires relaxation, such as a sunset or the ocean.

Massage: Massage has been demonstrated to be very effective during pregnancy. It has been shown to decrease depression, leg and back pains, and anxiety during labour. A good massage may decrease the amount of cortisol (a stress hormone) in the body and help promote better relaxation. Studies have even showed that women who were massaged by their partner every 15 minutes during labour actually reduced their labour time by 3 hours! The best position for a labour massage is to be bent over the side of a bed or on all fours, so your partner can press firmly on the bottom of your back and on both sides of your hips. This is known to reduce back pain, especially for women who are suffering mainly from back labour. Using a lightly scented lotion or oil may also be more comforting for mom.

Aromatherapy: Some birthing centres and hospitals allow a light scent in the delivery room from putting a few drops of essential oils on the pillows or hospital bed. The scent of lavender is known to relax the mind and body and can be very useful in calming the body during labour. Other relaxation scents that can be used are vanilla, cocoa butter, or flower aromas.

Swaying: This is a technique recommended by midwives to help reduce back and hip pain and to progress labour. The mother sits on a birthing ball and rolls her hips in a circular motion or side to side. This helps relieve the pressure of the baby on the uterus. If a birthing ball is unavailable, holding on to a table or the side of a bed and gently rocking the hips from side to side in a swaying motion can also help reduce the pain and help progress labour by allowing gravity to move the baby lower and lower.

All fours: There are many positions a woman can try while in labour, such as lying on her back or side. However, many women say that the most relaxing and comfortable position is when they are balancing on their hands and knees. Being on all fours will take a lot of pressure off your back and hips and can sometimes ease contractions. This is also a perfect position for your partner to step in and give you a relaxing massage to help you get through the pain of contractions.

Water: Whether or not you are planning on having a water birth, having a birthing tub or shower can be a great idea. Warm water on the skin can ease labour pains and help the body to relax. Usually every hospital room has a private shower with a chair inside so the mother can sit down and have the warm water from the showerhead running on her back and belly. Moms who deliver their baby using the water birth method have insisted that it does help them cope with the pain. Getting in and out of the water from time to time during contractions has been found to be very beneficial. The more relaxed the body is, the easier labour will be.

TENS machine: TENS machines are commonly used during the early stages of labour as a replacement for pain medication. TENS stands for transcutaneous electrical nerve stimulation. A TENS machine is a small box consisting of one or two cords connected by wires to sticky pads that go directly onto the skin (usually on the lower back or hips of the pregnant woman). The machine gives out little pulses of electrical energy. You can purchase a TENS machine at a physiotherapy equipment store, some pharmacies, or online. Although this may not decrease the amount of pain you are feeling, it stimulates the nerves to distract you during contractions.

Laughing gas: Laughing gas is another non-medical option that some women would rather use in place of having an epidural. Although some women consider this not to be natural, the gas you breath in does not affect your baby in the least bit and is completely safe for mother as well. Most of all, it's controlled by the mother. You take it when you need it, rather than having an epidural that induces numbness until it wears off. Laughing gas is nothing more than nitrous oxide. It is super easy to administer and can be effective in less than a minute. It is known to take away the hard edges of the pain, allowing for the mother to feel more relief.

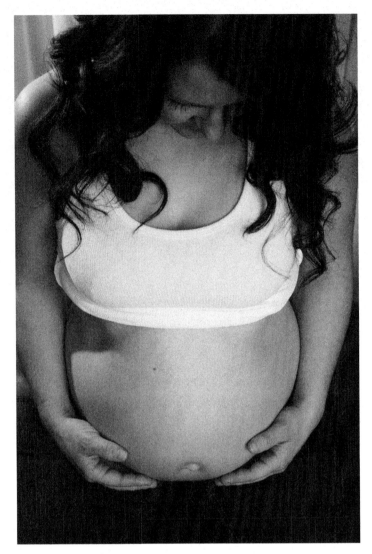

You come first photography

So mothers, no need to worry about going into labour with no methods to use for pain management. All of these suggestions are completely natural and quite effective. Just remember, no one can tell you which method will work for you and which one to use. It is up to you to use your judgment while in labour and find a method that works best for you. You may find that none of these methods work for your body, but when you are in labour you may hit upon a technique that works perfectly for you, even if no one has ever heard of it. Your body is intelligent and will tell you exactly what it likes and what it doesn't.

Some women have to try several techniques before finding the right one, and sometimes one will work for the first stage but not for the second. Play around and listen to your body for the best pain management and relaxation technique. What you are going through is only temporary and will eventually come to an end. However, what you will get out of it will last forever, so don't give up!

Push it, push it real good!

Now that you have overcome the labour pains and contractions, the next stage of labour is pushing time! During this time, it is important to get in your most comfortable position. So try a number of different positions, until you find one that you feel the most comfortable in. Don't worry, you don't HAVE to be on your back. It may be easier for your doctor to deliver when you are lying on your back with your legs spread apart, but this may not be the best and most comfortable way for you to push your baby out. In fact, most woman find this to be the most painful and unnatural way of giving birth as lying on your back doesn't allow you to work with gravity. Rather than opening up the hips and allowing for the birth canal to open, you're putting pressure on the uterus and causing blockage. This means more pushing and more time is needed to get the baby out. Giving birth lying on your back can also lead to unnecessary interventions like tearing, an episiotomy, forceps delivery, or a vacuum extraction.

Here are five different birth positions to try, which may make your baby's delivery faster and easier. These positions can be used for the first stages of labour as well as the second stage and active labour.

1. Sitting positions: Sitting positions combine relaxation with the force of gravity, allowing for a more open passage for the baby to easily make his/her way down the birth canal. A birth ball, rocking, or toilet sitting are often used as a resting tool, while the pressure of gravity helps labour progress.

2. Squatting positions: By engaging the body in a squatting position during labour, you are allowing for the pelvis to open and the baby to find an optimal position for birth. Squatting throughout your whole labour and pushing phase may become extremely exhausting, so rely on the support of your partner or a squatting bar. Many hospitals and birth centres will have these on hand.

3. Hands and knees position: There are two specific positions that involve being on all fours: the full moon and the crawl. These positions are excellent for reducing back labour, turning a posterior baby, and maybe even when delivering a larger baby.

4. Side-lying positions: During the long and tiring hours of labour, side-lying positions are great for resting in-between contractions. This position promotes a body-wide relaxation and minimizes the effort of self-stabilization. Because gravity isn't working at its best during this position, it is best used in the later stages of labour.

5. Upright or standing positions: This is the one position that uses the greatest amount of gravity during the birthing stage. It allows the baby to drop into the pelvis and prevents pressure from concentrating in one spot. Less than 5% of women use this position when delivering their baby, aside from all of its benefits.

Just like when choosing the right method of relaxation and natural pain relief methods during labour, not every position works for everyone. You may want to try all or a few of these positions until you find out the one that's most comfortable for you. It is very rare that a woman will find one position that suits her for her entire labour and delivery, so don't be alarmed if you have to switch it up plenty of times before you settle in to deliver your child.

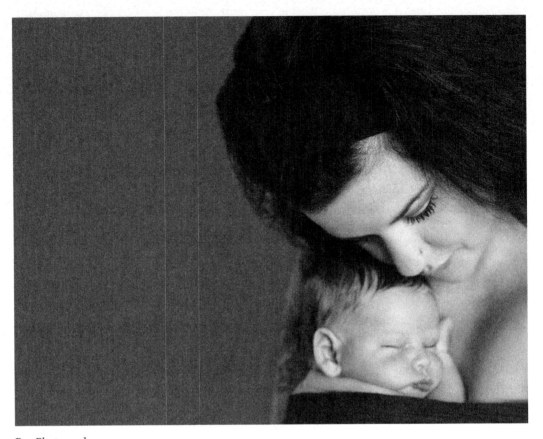

Pop Photography

Chapter 9
Welcome Baby

Well moms, congratulations, you did it! Whether or not your birthing experience went exactly as planned or completely the opposite, you now have your little angel in your arms. Without words, he or she is thanking you for providing him or her with the love, nurturing, and care you delivered throughout your pregnancy.

So now what? You've managed to push through the 9 months of this miraculous journey, only to find out there are many questions and obstacles you must face after pregnancy. Besides the obvious lack of sleep, an overload of dirty diapers and bibs, spit-up all over your new blouse, and still looking like you are 6 months pregnant after you have delivered baby, what are the necessary steps you must take in order to nourish your child as he or she moves through the different stages of life.

Breastfeeding

Is breast the best?

Now that your little one is born, you've probably thought already about what feeding method to use to nourish your child. Breast milk or formula? While this decision may be easy for some moms, other moms wonder what the best choice is and how they can decide.

I've narrowed down some excellent points when it comes to breast milk versus formula and how this decision can be decided, if not already.

According to the AAP (American Academic of Pediatrics), mothers should breastfeed their babies for up to 6 months minimum. From my research and personal opinion, a mother should feed her child breast milk for as long as possible, or until the child wishes to no longer take it. Some mothers chose to breastfeed until the child is one or two and the world's average for the latest age for breastfeeding was 4 years! Some people would be shocked if a mother were to them that they were still breastfeeding their child (most likely pumping, due to the full mouth of teeth!)

at the age of 4. This is completely safe and super healthy for the child, as breast milk contains so many essential nutrients that provide the child's body and brain with everything it needs to grow. It's even healthy for the mothers! But I'll get more into this later...

Although the experts recommend breastfeeding as the exclusive first food for babies, it may not be possible for all mothers. It can be based on their comfort level, lifestyle, and even certain medical issues. So when is it unsafe for mothers to breastfeed? The answer is if you:

- Are infected with the human immunodeficiency virus (HIV)
- Are taking antiretroviral medications
- Have untreated, active tuberculosis
- Are infected with human T-cell lymphotropic virus type I or type II
- Are using or are dependent upon illegal drugs
- Are dependent on alcohol
- Are taking prescribed cancer chemotherapy agents, such as antimetabolites that interfere with DNA replication and cell division
- Are undergoing specific radiation therapies

So whether or not you chose to or not to breastfeed, don't ever feel guilty about your decision, especially if it is something you simply cannot do. If you can and chose to breastfeed, you are providing your baby with so many health benefits, as well as strengthening the mother and baby bond.

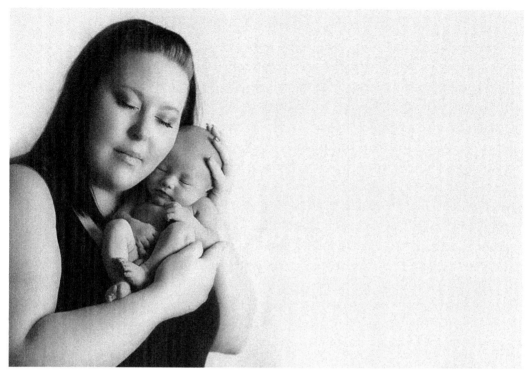

Pop Photography

Benefits of breastfeeding

Here are some of the many benefits of breastfeeding your baby:

1. Breast milk helps reduce and fight infection, such as ear and respiratory infections, meningitis and diarrhea. Breast milk also contributes to strengthening your baby's immune system by increasing the barriers to infection and decreasing the growth of bacteria and other viral organisms.

2. Breastfeeding has been known to show benefits in premature babies and have a number of protective components that can benefit your child later in life, as well as help prevent allergies, diabetes, asthma, obesity, and SIDS.

3. Breast milk is also known as the perfect food for infants. It is specifically designed by the body for the body, especially for a newborn's digestive system. The components of breast milk are easily digested by the newborn's delicate and immature digestive system. Having a healthy digestive system decreases and even eliminates the chances of diarrhea and constipation.

Essentials in breast milk

Another benefit of breast milk, which I consider to be the most important one, is its nutrient content! Let's take a look at what ingredients are present in this perfectly balanced meal.

High-quality protein: Although human milk is much lower in protein than other mammal milk like cow's or goat's milk, there is some logic behind it. Mother's milk contains low amounts of high-quality protein, because the human baby is designed to grow slowly, compared to a calf that doubles its birth weight in less than three months. The higher the level of protein, the faster and the larger our babies would grow in a shorter amount of time, and I don't know if any mom wants that just yet. Although this wonderful liquid gold, as some would call it, is low in proteins, it contains all the essential amino acids, which are the building blocks of protein. In particular, breast milk has a very high level of the essential amino acid, taurine. This amino acid is primarily responsible for the development of the baby's brain and eyes.

Calcium: Be aware that some infants, especially if inherited from the mother, are lactose intolerant, which means their little digestive systems cannot properly digest the sugar in milk. It is extremely important that mothers who are breastfeeding lactose intolerant babies stay away from any dairy products themselves, as the lactose can be passed into the breast milk and absorbed by the baby. Monitor your baby for any signs and symptoms of gas, bloating, colic, constipation, and/or diarrhea, as these may be symptoms that your baby is not properly digesting lactose.

Mothers may consume dairy alternatives to ensure their baby will not have to suffer from the symptoms of a lactose sensitivity or allergy. Organic goat's milk and/or fortified almond and rice milks make great dairy replacements and do contain a certain amount of calcium. A daily calcium supplement is highly recommended, even if the mother is consuming regular cow's milk. Calcium is an extremely important nutrient in infants and is responsible for their growth and the strength and health of their bones.

Ah! My absolute favourite ingredient, FAT: Breast milk is made up of almost all fat, and not just any fat, but a very good source of fast-digesting fats, which leads to better absorption into the bloodstream. Not only is the fat in breast milk easily digested, it is also the healthy fat and contains DHA, AA, and cholesterol – the fats that are vital to our health.

Human milk also contains high amounts of linoleic and linoleic acid. These fatty acids contribute to the development of myelin, a substance that covers the nerves and assists the nerves in transmitting messages to other nerves throughout the brain and body.

The fat in breast milk is an excellent source of energy for growing babies and is also very essential to the development of the brain, as the brain is made up mostly of fat. The lack of fats in an infant's diet can lead to an abundance of problems.

Fats are very important in the development of the retinal and nervous system development. Symptoms such as poor growth, degenerative changes in internal organs, dysfunctional vision, and slow brain development can result in fat deficiencies. A low intake of fats may also increase the chances of children developing behavioral and learning problems such as ADHD. Some studies have even shown a correlation between essential fatty acid deficiency and autism. Many, if not all, of these complications can be prevented by providing your baby with good quality breast milk, as fat is its middle name!

Breast milk is extremely nutrient dense and contains every essential vitamin and mineral our growing baby needs. Not only does human milk contain much higher amounts of these vitamins and minerals compared to the added nutrients in formula, the vitamins and minerals in breast milk are also much easier to absorb.

According to Dr. Donald Rudin, author of the book The Omega 3 Phenomenon, "There is no comparable substitute for the remarkable mix of nutrients and immunity-boosting factors provided by mother's milk, as long as the mother is eating properly. A well-nourished nursing mother provides her infant with a perfect blend of essential fatty acids and their long-chained derivatives, assuring the fast-growing brain and body tissues a rich supply. Mother's milk also supplies important antibodies not present in cow's milk or in artificial formula."

Essentials in breast milk

These essential vitamins are present in breast milk:

1. Vitamin A: This is very high in colostrum, which is the first milk that comes out of the breast. It appears to be more yellowish than white and is the highest nutrient containing food for a newborn baby. This is what the mother produces before her actual milk supply comes in.

2. Vitamin D: Since breast milk contains a very small amount of this vitamin, it is recommended that breastfeeding women take an additional vitamin D supplement, especially if they are living somewhere that sunlight is not always present.

3. Vitamin E: There is also a very high amount of this in colostrum. Vitamin E is an excellent antioxidant and can also help prevent hemolytic anemia.

4. Vitamin K: This vitamin is very beneficial in preventing hemorrhagic disease in a newborn. Hemorrhagic disease is a clotting or bleeding disorder in a newborn, due to a vitamin K deficiency. This is why all babies are given a shot of vitamin K right after birth.

5. Vitamin C: This powerful antioxidant can also help in strengthening the immune system. Vitamin C may benefit the mother as well by increasing her milk supply.

6. B complex: This includes thiamine, riboflavin, niacin, pantothenic acid, B6, folic acid, and B12. B vitamins are mainly responsible for assisting the body to metabolize the macronutrients (carbohydrates, fats, and proteins) in foods.

7. Prebiotics and probiotics: Prebiotics are a non-digestible source of carbohydrates that assist in balancing the intestinal microorganisms or flora by stimulating the growth of probiotics. The probiotic strain bifido bacteria are also commonly found in breast milk, which helps to develop a healthy immune system in infants.

What to include in your diet while nursing

There are certain vitamins and minerals that you should take in on a daily basis and which can become a particular concern during breastfeeding.

1. Protein: A breastfeeding mother needs more protein now than she did while she was pregnant. Not by much, but now that you are breastfeeding, you should be consuming around 67 grams of protein a day. You can find protein in sources like fish, chicken and turkey breast, eggs, legumes, lean red meat, and whole grains, as well as in supplements such as natural vegan protein powder.

2. Folate: This vitamin is one of the most important vitamins during pregnancy and breastfeeding, as this is the B vitamin required for the growth and development of your child. You should be taking about 450 to 500 IU of folic acid per day. High amounts of folate can be found in leafy green vegetables, oranges, whole grains, and some nuts and seeds.

3. Vitamin A: This is essential for normal growth, healthy vision, and the prevention of infections. It is recommended that a breastfeeding mother consume 800 to 1200 IU daily. Vitamin A is also found in egg yolks, liver, fatty fish, carrots, and other orange and green vegetables.

4. Calcium: Nursing mothers need to be very careful about their intake of calcium, as it is an extremely important nutrient. Moms who are nursing should aim for 1000 mg of calcium daily. Studies show that breastfeeding women can often lose 3 to 5 percent of their bone mass when breastfeeding if calcium intake is not sufficient.

To ensure that you are getting the recommended dosage of the necessary nutrients while breastfeeding, continue to take a prenatal vitamin and consume a whole-foods diet with plenty of variety.

What to avoid while nursing

As much as there are great things to eat while nursing, there are a few substances that should only be consumed in moderation. These include:

1. Caffeine: Now that your baby is out, you are probably thinking, "YES! Coffee and tea again, no more sleepiness from those 3am wake-up calls." As much as you're looking forward to your 4 cups of coffee a day, caffeine still needs to be limited while nursing. Caffeine can be absorbed into your breast milk and transferred to your baby during feeding. Moms who consume excessive caffeine report that their babies feel jittery and irritable, develop sleep problems, and sometimes even become constipated. This is because your baby's body cannot tolerate that much caffeine at such a young age. Caffeine can also disrupt milk production

and affect the nutritional value of the milk. Caffeine should be limited to a minimum of 2 cups per day to prevent any of the concerns listed above from caffeine consumption.

2. Alcohol: This substance can affect breast milk even more than caffeine. Having a drink once in a while is not considered harmful. But if you do have an occasional beer or glass of wine, be sure you wait at least 2 to 4 hours before breastfeeding or have milk pumped beforehand and then proceed to "pump and dump" right after consuming alcohol. Not drinking in general is the safest option while breastfeeding.

3. Certain foods: There are some foods that can be irritating to your baby if eaten on a regular basis while nursing. Some babies experience gas, bloating, constipation, and colic when mothers eat certain foods. Spicy foods and vegetables such as cabbage and broccoli may affect your baby's belly, so watch for signs of discomfort. If your baby displays any symptoms, stop eating those foods and watch if it makes a difference. Once you see that your baby's symptoms have disappeared, try introducing that food back into your diet. If the symptoms arise again, it's best to avoid that food as much as possible during the remaining nursing period.

A common question my clients ask me about is how long they should breastfeed for. In my personal opinion, the longer one breastfeeds, the better. Most health professionals say that a baby should receive breast milk for a minimum of 6 months and then be supplemented with formula up until one year of age. According to the World Health Organization (WHO), babies should be breastfed for at least 2 years. This does not mean exclusively breastfeeding, but nursing at least once a day to supplement a healthy diet already consisting mainly of solid foods.

Breast milk is extremely healthy and full of essential nutrients, so the longer you breastfeed, the less likely it is that your baby will become infected with an illness. If you plan on breastfeeding for longer than 6 months, solid foods should still be introduced at the appropriate time, as a child cannot rely fully on breast milk after the age of 6 months.

So the ultimate decision is yours. Just know that if you do wish to breastfeed for a longer period of time, pumping may be an option to consider versus strict baby-to-breast feeding. Teeth usually begin to develop around 6 to 8 months, and if you don't want to risk getting bitten by your little guy, pumping your milk and bottle-feeding may be the best way to go.

Colic

Oh, Colic, how we despise you. As a mother, this has been one of the hardest things to deal with. And as a parent who has or is currently experiencing colic with their infant, you may feel the same way. Seeing a baby in discomfort and pain is hard for anyone, but thankfully, mothers, doctors, and geniuses alike, have came up with many, wonderful, natural treatments for colicky infants.

What is colic?

Colic is described as uncontrollable crying in a healthy infant. No matter what you do, colic may seem like the impossible when trying to calm your child. If your infant is about 4 months or younger and continuously cries for periods of 2 to 3 hours in a row or seems like he/she is always unhappy and in discomfort, your child is considered to be "colicky". Colic is quite common and is said to affect roughly 20 percent of babies in their first few months of life. Don't worry mamas, colic is not dangerous and will not affect your baby's growth or development in anyway.

Most newborn will cry, some more than others, but as a parent you will learn the difference between cries of hunger, poop, sleepiness, and colic! Colic will stand out like a sore thumb, and as mentioned above, it will continue for quite a while, with nothing stopping it. Some mothers describe colic as a "crying attack" caused by some sort of stomach pain.

For mothers who have infants dealing with colic, you have to always remember that it is not your fault, and you are never doing anything wrong. Colic is simply out of your control and will pass eventually.

Causes

Although there may be no one cause for colic, it appears that colic is associated with a pain in the abdomen connected with indigestion. Others suspect colic when their infants are going through that phase of spitting up after each feeding. If you feel like your child is "colicky", no matter what their exact symptoms are, just stay positive and do your best to cope and help your little one cope as well.

So how is it that if there is no exact definition of colic that we know if an infant is actually colicky? Here are the commonly displayed symptoms of children with colic. If a good percent of them match up with what your child seems to be experiencing, your child can be considered colicky, and you can look into ways to treat it naturally.

1. Babies tend to cry for no reason, and all babies cry at some points throughout the day. But colicky babies seem to cry for no specific reason, and their crying can last quite a while, with no method of comfort seeming to calm them down.

2. Colicky babies may have a specific time of day when they tend to cry for no reason. It could be in the morning upon rising or before they go to bed. You may start to see a pattern that could indicate your baby has colic.

3. The three 3's: They cry for more than 3 hours at a time. They cry for more than 3 days a week, and they cry for about 3 weeks. This is a generic guideline when it comes to judging whether or not your infant is colicky.

4. Their pitch of cry is much different than usual. It can be louder and higher pitched than normal.

5. Babies with colic have a very hard time being soothed, no matter what you do. Rocking, singing, nursing, and swaddling do nothing to stop them from crying.

6. You have an overall healthy baby, and your baby displays no problems throughout the day.

7. Your baby has a very hard belly and may even start to bend his/her knees into his/her belly as a sign of discomfort.

8. Your baby shows signs of gassiness, especially when crying episodes occur. (This is where the bicycle legs movement comes in handy!)

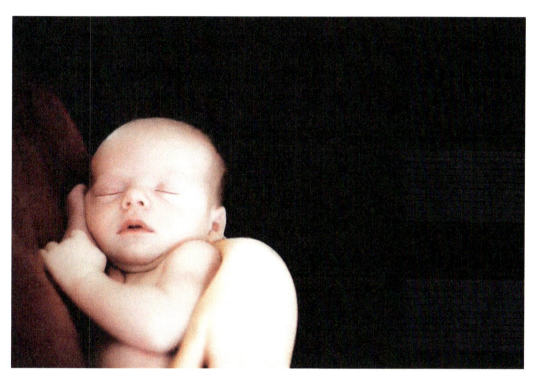

JM Photography

Coping

Some babies are different and may be much harder to calm when they are experiencing colic, but here are some natural ways that you can try to sooth them when they are experiencing an outburst:

1. Massage: Belly massages may help soothe your baby by helping him/her to pass any gas he/she may be struggling to release. Using gently scented essential oils such as lavender, echinacea, and candeluna may also help your baby to relax. You may even try gently placing your baby on his/her stomach and rubbing his/her back.

2. Burping: Make sure after each feeding, you burb your baby completely. It may take a little time before you get a good burp out, but it's worth it if that's what it takes to soothe your little one. You can even try burping half way through the feeding to let out any gas that has already started to build up.

3. Assess your diet: In a lot of cases when I work with mothers who have concerns about a colicky baby, I notice that there are certain foods in their diet that may be responsible for their baby's colic. Soon enough after removing these foods from their diet (until the nursing period is over), their baby's colic has completely cleared. Some of the top foods that can irritate a baby are: potent spices such as curries or chili; citrus fruits such as oranges, lemons, limes, and grapefruit; all dairy products (as baby may have a sensitivity); caffeine (including chocolate as it contains high amounts); gluten and soy.

4. For bottle-feeding moms, switch up their formula: This goes for constipated babies as well as for colicky ones. If your infant is strictly on a cow's milk formula, try using an alternative like goat's milk (do not use soy). Some mothers have even found that organic cow's milk formula is gentler on tummies and has helped eased colic. (Organic cow's milk formula does not contain some of the added ingredients given to cows to prevent illness and promote a larger milk supply.) Other moms have even made their own formula using Dr. Westin Price's formula.

5. Different brands of formula, even if they are all dairy, may affect your baby's colic differently. Try alternating between two different brands and see if that type of formula rotation helps reduce your infant's colic symptoms.

6. Bottle rotation or using a different bottle: Alternating from one bottle to another may help reduce colic symptoms in your infant as the flow can differ from bottle to bottle. Another great option is to find a bottle that is designed for the reduction of colic. These bottles tend to be more expensive as they usually come equipped with built-in airflow or ventilation and a nipple built for a slower milk flow. Look for bottles that say they mimic the breast or nursing. This will ensure that less air is inhaled by your baby, therefore reducing colic

7. Homeopathic remedies: My own son experienced horrible colic, even though he was nursing and only bottle-fed on occasion. I was the desperate mother who tried everything and nothing worked. Luckily for me, I was recommended a homeopathic formula that would make life so much easier. Although there are plenty of great natural remedies on the market, I truly value a brand called Boiron and their product Cocyntal, which is exclusively designed to help reduce colic. Feel free to do your own research and find a brand that works best for your child, as every child is unique. I highly recommend if none of the other natural remedies work to soothe your child, try a homeopathic remedy, usually found in a liquid form, before having to resort to a visit to the doctor's office.

8. Probiotics: As will be mentioned under infant supplements, probiotics have been shown to reduce colic symptoms significantly.

Chapter 10
Boobs and Barbells

Nursing and exercise

Now that your baby is being taken care of with a healthy diet and much love from mum and dad, you've probably been thinking a little bit about yourself and wondering when your baby weight is going to come off. In fact, right after giving birth, you may have already lost anywhere from 10 to 15 pounds(4.5 to 6kg), as some of the weight you put on wasn't fat, but weight from extra blood and fluid retention, breast tissue, the placenta, and of course, your baby!

The key to losing your baby weight and keeping it off without affecting your health, energy, and milk supply (if you are breastfeeding) is patience and time. Think about it. It took you 9 months to gain all the necessary and sometimes unnecessary weight for your baby. It could take just as long to get back to pre-pregnancy weight. If you've gained more then the recommended pregnancy weight gain, understand that it will most likely take a bit longer to shed those extra pounds than if you had gained the recommended 25 to 35 pounds(11-15kg)

You should be happy to know many moms eventually drop below their pre-pregnancy weight if eating properly and exercising! All you have to do is find a good routine that you are happy with and can do consistently.

Food first

First things first. You need to continue the routine of healthy eating and filling up on healthy, low-calorie, high-density, nutritious foods, just like you did doing pre-conception and your pregnancy. Thankfully, your pregnancy cravings should have decreased now that your hormones are balancing out.

Diet is 80 percent responsible for a healthy weight composition. Fifteen percent is exercise and five percent is genetics. So yes, diet is a huge, if not the most important, factor that contributes to your weight. It is also a very important aspect when trying to keep your body energized and healthy and in allowing your body to heal faster from the effects of childbirth.

Moms will admit that after their child is born, it is hard to find the time or energy to get back into a consistent physical activity routine. Exercise is necessary and will benefit you even more when combined with a healthy diet. So if you are the one who struggles in the beginning because of a lack of sleep and wanting to spend all your time with your new family member, a healthy diet is the way to begin your journey to shedding those pounds!

Let's keep in mind though, mamas, that extreme dieting is not an option at this point, especially if you're breastfeeding. Breastfeeding moms do have the benefit of getting back to their pre-pregnancy weight quicker than formula-feeding moms, but they also require extra calories to keep up their milk supply and provide additional energy for themselves. Breastfeeding burns anywhere from 250 to 500 calories a day, so it is recommended that a mother consume an additional 250 to 500 calories a day on top of what she needs to maintain her pre-pregnancy weight.

Nursing mothers will also feel that their hunger is over the top! What happened to the thought of our normal appetites returning after childbirth? Well, when your body is burning that many calories from producing food for your little one, you are going to need to feed yourself more food more often to keep up that supply and demand for your milk. So don't worry breastfeeding moms, you can still lose the weight while consuming additional calories, as long as those calories are coming from unprocessed foods! How cool is that? The more you breastfeed, the more calories your body burns making milk!

A good range for a breastfeeding mother to consume in calories is about 2000 to 2400 calories, with an additional 400 calories if you are feeding twins and 800 calories more if you are feeding triplets. A mother, regardless if she is breastfeeding or not, should not intake less than 1500 calories a day or she may be putting her health and milk supply at risk.

I absolutely hate the term "counting calories" as it is a waste of time and effort, but you do need to eat more quality foods. The key is not to count and add up every calorie you eat to ensure you are taking in the extra 400 to 500 calories, but rather to listen to your body and eat when you feel hungry. From my personal experience and that of my many clients who are currently nursing, it is usual to feel hungry every three hours, or sometimes every two, so stay attuned with your inner hunger and feed your body when you need it.

Hydration is another very important aspect when breastfeeding, as dehydration can lessen the milk supply. Drink as much pure spring or filtered water as possible, aiming for 10 to 12 glasses a day. Hydration will also help your body stay energized and will speed up your metabolism.

While breastfeeding, what you eat on a daily basis may not have a direct effect on the quality of your milk as whatever it lacks, it will take from your body and give it to your baby. So rather than your milk being low in certain nutrients, it will be your body that can suffer from malnutrition. Breast milk can take a lot from your body if your diet is not replenishing what the milk is talking, so nourish your body and make healthy choices that will benefit your health. How much you eat, on the other hand, can affect the quantity of your breast milk, which is why your caloric intake is so important.

For formula-feeding moms, you don't have to worry about adding those additional calories to your diet, and you will most likely not have an increase in appetite. Moms who choose not to breastfeed may wish to reduce their calorie intake to help increase weight loss, but be aware that your lack of sleep and having to tend to your newborn may leave you even more exhausted if your calorie intake is low. A 1500 calorie intake is the lowest we would recommend for these moms. Anything lower can put your body at risk of entering a starvation mode, in which losing weight will be harder and take much longer, since your body will be storing fat to sustain your life.

A better way to look at losing weight, rather than counting calories, is to focus on high-quality, unrefined and unprocessed, whole foods. Cut out all sugars and overly fatty foods, and focus more on whole grains, raw and steamed vegetables, fresh fruit, and healthy fats. In my studies and research as a holistic nutritionist, what I have seen work best for my clients seeking to lose weight is opting for a primarily vegetarian diet and excluding the diary products like milk and cheese, as well as gluten products, such as bread and pasta. These two foods are extremely difficult for the body to digest. They put a damper on your weight loss as the energy used to burn fat is now used to try and digest this unwanted food product.

Some mothers also worry about calcium intake as they are no longer consuming dairy, but have no fear. As long as you are consuming plenty of fresh, dark leafy greens and other green vegetables, along with raw nuts and seeds (such as sesame, which has a much higher content of calcium than milk), you will be completely safe. A calcium supplement is again available if you need that extra security, and especially for breastfeeding moms, this isn't a bad option to consider.

Eating an abundance of raw foods will also boost your weight loss, as they are very easy for the body to breakdown and digest. So aim for as much raw fruits and vegetables as you can, but be sure that you chose organic whenever possible.

Animal proteins can also be harder on the body to digest, as they can remain in the colon for up to 72 hours before leaving the body. This can cause the protein to rot and release toxins, making it much harder to lose weight. If you do not wish to opt for a fully vegetarian lifestyle, I recommend a digestive enzyme before your meal that contains animal protein. Consuming more easily digestible animal protein such as organic eggs and wild fish is a more ideal choice than consuming red meat.

Try to decrease the amount of animal proteins you eat by at least 3 times a week, if this seems possible. You should aim to eat vegetarian at least 4 times a week for more efficient and more sustainable weight loss.

Food choices and hydration are still just as important if you are using formula opposed to breast milk. Even if you are not ingesting as much as the breastfeeding mom, the quality of food you eat should be identical.

Holistic Food Guide

Consuming an array of whole foods should help you get back into shape while still giving your baby all the essential nutrients! Every meal should contain one of the following food groups to create a balanced, healthy meal.

Top whole grains and starches (1/2 cup to 1 cup serving, based on your caloric needs):
- Oats
- Barley
- Brown or wild rice
- Yams
- Potatoes
- Corn
- Quinoa
- Gluten-free bread or wraps
- Winter or butternut squash
- Amaranth
- Buckwheat
- Wheatberry
- Bulgur
- Rye
- Spelt

Proteins (organic and free-range whenever possible):
- Chicken breast
- Turkey breast
- All legumes (beans, lentils)
- Tofu (limit as it is a soy product)
- Light tuna
- Wild Salmon and other fatty fish
- Sole, tilapia, cod, haddock, and other white fish
- All raw nuts and seeds
- Whole grains
- Eggs
- All natural vegan protein powders
- Plain, unsweetened goat yogurt
- Plain coconut or almond yogurt

Fibrous carbohydrates (1 serving of fruit, unlimited vegetables):
- Oranges
- Apples
- Grapes

- Melons
- Bananas
- Grapefruit
- Lemons and limes
- Berries (blue, black, strawberries, and raspberries)
- Spinach
- Asparagus
- Mixed bell peppers
- Broccoli
- Carrots
- Cucumber
- Romaine lettuce
- Kale
- Peas
- Cauliflower
- All fresh herbs

All fruits and vegetables are an excellent source of nutrients, so pile them high on your plate! Healthy fats (Use in moderation, 25 to 35 grams of fat a day is a good range):

- Avocado
- All raw nuts and seeds
- Olive and other non-processed vegetable oils
- Virgin coconut oil
- Egg yolk
- Raw or organic, full-fat milk and cheeses (if you choose to eat dairy)
- Almond milk
- Red meats

There are plenty other unique, whole food choices on the market today, aside from the ones listed. Be creative and go to your local farmers' market and fill up on a variety of these or other whole foods, but be sure they are organic! Pesticides and other chemicals can be absorbed into the breast milk and given to your baby, making him/her ill. By choosing organic, you are avoiding passing all of these harmful additives onto your precious baby!

Cleaning out your refrigerator and cupboard after pregnancy is a great way to kick back into your healthy eating habits, especially if you've slipped up during pregnancy. Having more healthy food choices around your house and less junk food will make it much easier to avoid those nasty cravings.

Moms who are breastfeeding and even moms who are choosing formula may be still going through hormonal changes. This means that those cravings you've been having during pregnancy may still linger for months after giving birth. Some professionals recommend not beginning any diet plans until 2 months after birth. You may be surprised that you still crave chocolate ice cream and gummy worms during the post-partum period, but don't fret, as these hormones and food cravings will calm eventually. As long as you are not overly indulging in these unhealthy cravings all the time, you can still safely shed your post-pregnancy weight while enjoying those occasional treats!

Exercise

Now that you've hopefully regained some energy back, you may be wondering when you can start back up in the exercise department. Although you may not want to at this point, engaging yourself in physical activity will benefit you more than you think.

It is important that before beginning any new or previous exercise regime that you get the okay from your doctor. If your pregnancy and birth went as planned with no complications, it may be safe for you to start as early as 4 weeks after giving birth. If you received a C-section or had a more traumatic birth experience, your doctor may want you to wait until the 6-week mark or until you are fully recovered before you begin to work out.

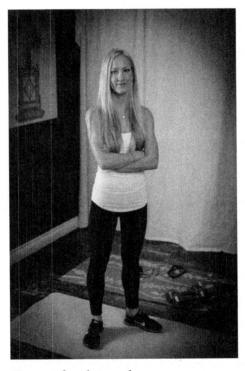

You come first photography

It is recommended that moms who are getting back into working out start off slowly. Gradually walking for 30 minutes every day, then moving up to 45 to 60 minutes a day, is a good way to start. Yoga is another low-intensity activity that's great to begin when getting back into shape after having your baby. There are even mommy and baby yoga classes, which you can do with your new baby and that are great for bonding. Once your body is warmed up and has begun getting used to being active on a more regular basis, you can start to pump up the intensity.

Weightlifting is an excellent, functional exercise that not only helps build up lean muscle mass, but also accelerates the fat-burning process. Some mothers may have been unfortunate enough to not have been able to be physically active while pregnant, either due to a high-risk, bed-rest pregnancy, constant morning sickness, or extreme fatigue. In these cases, a lot of precious muscle mass is lost due to the lack of movement, so weightlifting on a weekly basis will help build that muscle mass and strength back up. Weightlifting also increases your metabolism, therefore, allowing the body to burn more fat!

Start off slowly, especially if you've never lifted weights before. Begin with lighter weights and more repetitions. Eventually build up to heavier weights and fewer repetitions and mix in some cardio to transform your body into a fat-burning machine. Weightlifting can also increase your energy! And we all know that new moms are going to need more energy than anyone at this point!

Some new moms insist that hiring a personal trainer to get them back into shape or at least to get them started is the best way to go, especially if they are completely new to exercise. A personal trainer can get you on the right path and customize a routine specifically for your goals. Some gyms even have a small day care centre included in their facility, so you can do your work out and be around your child at the same time. If you are one of those moms who doesn't wish to go all the way to a gym to get a good work out, why not invest in a couple sets of dumbbells. You don't even need to go out and purchase any cardio equipment if you live near a pathway and the weather is decent most of the year. Even purchasing a few home workout DVD's can give you the benefit of a great workout without leaving the comfort of your own home.

Balancing out your life with some cardio, weightlifting, healthy eating, and enough rest will get your pre-pregnancy body back (or even better!), while allowing you and your family to live a healthy lifestyle.

So give it time, new mommies, and you will eventually get to where you want to be. Be patient and give yourself enough credit. You're a new mom now, and your baby is now your number one priority, but this should never be an excuse to give up on keeping yourself healthy and happy! Stay confident in yourself with a positive mindframe and always remember, consistency is the key!

Chapter 11
Moving On Up From Milk

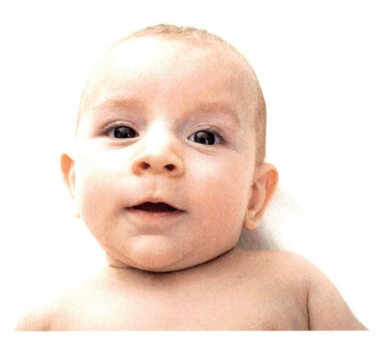

You come first photography

Ah! The moment so many of you have been waiting for! The introduction to solid foods! Personally, as a new mother, this was one of my favourite moments in my infant's growing life. I was looking forward to all the new tastes and meal ideas I could whip up and test on my, hopefully, not-too-much-of-a-picky-eater, baby!

Maybe it's just me, but making my own nutritious food combinations from local, organic, whole foods just made the experience that much better. I love being in the kitchen cooking for others and myself, and I got to take on a whole new approach to cooking for my little one.

A baby's first solid feeding is such a crucial step in his/her life, as this is where he/she is finally being introduced to everyday food – not just mama's milk or formula – but food he/she will be eating on an everyday basis for the rest of his/her life. Why is this so important you may ask? Once a child's palate is developed, they are most likely going to base their day-to-day food choices on foods that rotate around what their palates have become accustomed to.

If you only feed your infant green beans and yogurt because those are the only foods he or she seems to enjoy or even keep down, you may be setting yourself up for a hard run in the future when it comes to trying new foods and eating healthy food choices.

It's important to introduce a wide variety of infant-suitable foods to your child's growing palate at a young age. This will result in healthier eaters, and less picky eaters, which you moms will thank me for in the future. It also allows them to be independent and to choose from different options based on their own cravings and nutritional needs. It also makes the whole "you are eating what I make you or nothing at all" sessions so much easier.

When to begin

Most parents and doctors recommend beginning to introduce solid food to infants around 6 months of age. Some parents start a little earlier, while others a little later. This all depends on if your child is actually ready to begin eating solids. So how exactly do we know if our child is ready, as every child is different?

Here are some key points to watch out for in your little one, which can help determine if now is a good starting point to add solid foods. We don't want to push infants who may not be ready for solids as their digestive tract may not be quite mature enough to handle these new food sources, and this could lead to problems such as early food allergies and constipation or diarrhea. So go with your gut feeling, and if your child matches a majority of these signs, you should be okay to begin the introduction of solids to his/her diet.

1. Baby is sitting up well on their own, with limited support
2. You spot baby chewing on fingers or teething toys frequently
3. Baby's first teeth are appearing
4. Baby is eager to participate in mealtime and tries grabbing food from your plate or hands when he/she sees you eating
5. Baby has learned how to pick up small objects or food using his/her thumb and index finger together
6. Baby is 6 months old

As you can see, there are quite a few different signs that may show your baby's development has matured enough to start solids, and you can always switch back to all milk feedings if you find that your baby isn't ready yet and is having a hard time with these new foods.

As a mother, it is also highly recommend that you continue nursing, pumping, or supplementing with formula up until your baby is 1 year old. Nursing or formula feeding between solid meal times will allow your baby to still maintain all those powerful nutrients that they may not be obtaining from solid foods quite yet, especially the super important, healthy fatty acids!

Feeding time and first foods

A good rule is to start your baby on one new food per week, about one feeding per day, and working your way up to three feedings a day once your baby is comfortable and has tried a variety of new food. It is crucial to only start by trying one new food a week to help make it easier to spot any food allergies. When trying a new food every week, you can easily learn which specific food your baby cannot tolerate and remove it from their diet to try at a later time or remove completely if it a serious allergen. Trying a few foods per week may make it harder to point out exactly which food is causing a reaction.

Once you have gone through the list of all possible safe food choices for baby, you may start increasing the amount of feeds through the day and begin more of a variety of foods in one day.

Although there is still some controversy over whether it is better to start with a rice cereal or pureed, strained veggies and fruit, I do believe that our little one's digestive tracts are far to immature and delicate to start breaking down and absorbing grains, especially ones containing wheat!

I have worked with a lot of moms who started their infants on cereal products as a first food, then after dealing with constipation, upset and gassy stomachs, and colic, decided to downgrade the grains and replace with them with organic pureed fruits and vegetables. After they did this, they noticed that the symptoms of digestive discomfort were reduced significantly or disappeared.

Fruit and vegetables, especially organic ones, contain so many nutrients that are much easier digested and absorbed then grains. I am not saying to never give your child grains, just put them on hold until your child's digestive tract is more mature, usually around 1 year of age.

Feeding plan for baby

For those who have not yet begun solids, now is your chance to start feeding your baby the best foods from the start. You may choose to include some of the target foods on the allergen list such as dairy, but remember to avoid them if your baby shows symptoms.

Because your child's stomach is so sensitive and so small, we want to start with the easiest to digest and gentlest foods. I recommend starting your baby out with vegetables first versus fruits, as your child may prefer the sweetness of fruit and turn away when a vegetable comes to their mouth. Beginning with vegetables will give your child a fair chance to enjoy those tasty peas before being introduced to some juicy pears. You can then rotate between fruit and vegetables without a problem.

Best solid foods from age 6 months to 1 year

Babies 6 to 8 months old

Fruits: Avocado, peaches, pears, apples, bananas, plums, prunes, and pumpkin

Vegetables: Carrots, squash, peas, sweet potatoes or yams, green beans, zucchini

Organic meats: These may be introduced when baby is just starting on solids. However, I recommend waiting until about 8 months before introducing meat products, as starting with more gentle foods like fruits and vegetables gives your baby's stomach and digestive tract time to get use to digesting foods other than milk. The best meat choices are free-range chicken and turkey

Babies 8 to 11 months old

Fruits: Avocado, peaches, pears, apples, bananas, plums, prunes, pumpkin, cantaloupe, grapes, kiwi, mango, blueberries, cherries, papaya, dates, figs, watermelon, and honey-dew melon

Vegetables: Carrots, squash, peas, sweet potatoes or yams, green beans, zucchini, broccoli, asparagus, artichokes, cauliflower, onions, mushrooms, peppers, and eggplant

Proteins including meat products: Organic beef, free-range egg yolks, beans and legumes (lentils are the most easy to digest), and quinoa (which is a seed not a grain)

Dairy alternatives: Nut milks including coconut, brown rice milk, oat milk, coconut yogurt, non-dairy cheeses that do not contain soy and artificial ingredients. Another option is organic goat's milk. Although it does contain some lactose, it is much easier on the digestive system than cow's milk and contains less lactose than cow's milk.

Babies 12 months and up

At this age, your baby's digestive tract has built up more strength over the months, so he/she is able to tolerate a bigger variety of foods.

Fruits: Any fruits, including citrus (orange, lemons, grapefruit, limes), strawberries, raspberries, tomatoes, cucumbers

Vegetables: Any vegetables including organic corn, pickles

Proteins including meat products: Organic beef, turkey and chicken, wild fish, such as salmon, basa, sole, and other low mercury fish (keep an eye out for allergen symptoms as fish sensitivities are very common), whole free-range, organic eggs (whites and yolk)

Dairy-free alternatives: Nut milks including coconut, brown rice milk, oat milk, coconut yogurt, flax seed milk, non-dairy cheeses that do not contain soy and artificial ingredients, organic goat's milk and cheese, almond yogurt, homemade nut cheeses

Grains: Gluten-free oats, quinoa, millet, amaranth, buckwheat, gluten-free hard cereals (cheerios), gluten-free pasta, gluten-free breads and crackers, gluten-free cookies, brown rice

The more you introduce different foods and different textures when your child is young, the more expandable his/her palate will become, leading to a much less fussy eater in the future. Experiment with different recipes that include a variety of light spices and herbs, fresh smoothies with added greens, wild grains with mixed vegetables, and organic, homemade baking!

The Moo

Dairy is another common food that has been responsible for causing digestive symptoms in infants. Just like in adults, dairy acts as an acidifier in the body and is very hard to digest. Not just for those who suffer from lactose intolerance either. You can simply have a sensitivity to dairy rather than an allergy, but still end up having the same symptoms such as diarrhea, constipation, and gas.

It is recommended that dairy be avoided, not just in infancy but also through a child's life and into adulthood as the body does truly not need it. Unless you are currently supplementing your child's diet with a dairy-based supplement, no more dairy products should be added to their diet, even when formula supplementation is finished.

What about calcium? Do not fear mommies! Studies have found that plant-based calcium coming from leafy greens as well as some nuts and seeds like sesame contain even higher amounts of calcium than dairy. Research also shows that these sources of calcium are even more easily and efficiently digested and absorbed into the body, without having the consequences of dairy's acidity breaking down tissue in the bones.

As long as your child is eating a well-balanced diet with lots of greens, your calcium concerns are out the window, unless your child has a condition where more calcium is needed. There are many natural calcium supplements far better than dairy to satisfy those needs.

For those mothers who simply do not wish to give up diary, and that is truly okay as every parent's opinion can be different, I do recommend giving your child dairy products that can be much more easily digested than cow's milk. Goat's milk is a great alternative to cow's milk, contains higher levels of fat (which is essential for healthy brain development), and is much easier on the digestive system. There are even goat's milk formulas for infants who are lactose intolerant and do not wish to go on a soy-based supplement. Just ensure that if you are continuing or starting to introduce dairy-based products to your child's diet that they come from organic sources. There are far too many added chemicals in traditional on-the-shelf milk, which can seriously wreck havoc on your baby's health, especially when being introduced at such a young age.

Soy

I often get asked a lot of questions about soy-based formulas and soymilk as an alternative to dairy products. My answer is always, "I do not recommend soy, nor do I think it is a safe choice to give to babies, especially boys, at such a young age." Soy has an estrogenic effect on the body and is considered an estrogenic endocrine distributor by Dr. Mike Shelby, Director of CFSAN (Centre for Food Safety and Applied Nutrition). He states that many published studies show that consuming soy has negatively impacted developmental health, and during these precious developmental stages in your infant's life, the endocrine system should not be jeopardized.

Soy contains what are called "phytoestrogens". These phytoestrogens actually mimic the body's natural estrogen hormones. This can lead to a testosterone imbalance in boys, which is why males should avoid or drastically limit the amount of soy in their diet. For women, it can cause a drastic increase in estrogen, creating an estrogen dominance, which can cause infertility, cancer, and irregular menstrual cycles. Soy also contains lecithins, which can be harmful to the intestines.

If you still want to consider some soy products in your child's diet, aim for the unprocessed, organic, fermented soy products such as miso, gluten-free tamari sauce (aka soy sauce), and tempeh, a healthier substitute to tofu. As a large percent of soy products in North America are from genetically modified organisms (GMO), it is crucial to only consume organic soy products.

Dairy alternatives

With today's health culture rapidly growing, many other dairy alternatives have hit the market. But there are certain guidelines to follow, especially when giving these alternative dairy products to your infants.

First things first. None of these non-dairy milks should replace breast milk or formula at least until the first year of age, as they lack certain nutrients and fats that are essential to babies' growth and health. The second thing is food allergies. As some of these milks are nut-based, it is best to hold off on these beverages until the age of one in order to reduce the chance of developing or affecting any underlying allergies of which you may not be aware.

Once your child is over the age of one, it is then a safe time to start introducing non-dairy milks such as organic almond milk, flax seed milk, and other nut-based milks on the market. Be sure they come from organic, non-GMO sources, or even better, make them yourself! Homemade nut milks are one of the easiest things to make! You can find some wonderful recipes in the recipe section of this book.

If you want to introduce non-dairy, non-nut-based alternative milk products to your infant before the age of one, the three safest milks I recommend are brown rice milk, oat milk, and coconut milk (watch for coconut milk though as it's still considered a nut and may set off an allergic reaction in your child), which is less common than almond milk but is packed full of healthy saturated fatty acids!

Another important aspect you should look out for when choosing store-bought non-dairy milks is that they are UNSWEETENED. Sweetened beverages are usually loaded with sugars that your infant does not need. Unsweetened milks are very low in sugar, except for rice milks, which have a naturally higher sugar content.

Hydration

Now that we have covered the basics of what types of foods to feed babies who are just starting on solids, and some excellent dairy alternatives, it's very important to learn when it is best to hydrate your baby.

Most of society today is known to drink liquids with their meals, and this is a big NO NO! When we mix liquids such as water or juice with our solid meals, it really has a negative effect on our digestion and can lead to gas and a bloated and upset tummy, which leads to an unhappy baby.

When we begin to chew our food, our digestive stomach juices called hydrochloric acid begin stirring up to help break down and digest our food particles. But what happens when another liquid is being taken in along with food? The other beverage begins to dilute our hydrochloric acid, making it much harder to complete digestive tasks.

The best time to drink is in-between meals or 20 minutes before to 1 hour after. This gives the food enough time to breakdown and digest properly, ensuring your body is absorbing adequate amounts of nutrients.

Infant supplements

Most infants do not need supplements if they are eating a whole-foods diet and still consuming breast milk or formula daily. However, infant diets should be supplemented with vitamin D. Because they are not exposed to large amounts of sunlight and only a small amount of vitamin D is transferred in breast milk, supplementing 400 IU's, twice a day with infant vitamin D drops will ensure they will not become deficient. It is recommended that infants consume a vitamin D supplement from newborn to one year of age. In the months of October to April, supplementing your toddler with vitamin D isn't a bad idea especially if you live in an area that has longer winters.

Vitamin D will help prevent rickets as well as reduce the chance of illness in your baby's childhood. Rickets is a disease that causes the bones to soften and become frail and weak. This can result in bone deformities and fractures. Babies who are formula fed do not need the additional vitamin D supplement as they are getting the recommended dosage from formula.

Probiotics is also a wonderful supplement for infants and toddlers. As we know, having a healthy digestive system is the best way to prevent illness, as it is the first line of defense against compromised immunity. Probiotics are excellent for gastrointestinal health as they keep babies' intestinal flora healthy and vibrant. Boosting an infant's intestinal flora ensures he or she is absorbing the nutrients needed to grow and defend themselves against illness. A healthy gut equals a happy gut. In fact, studies have shown that supplementing infants' diets with probiotics significantly reduced their colic symptoms! When purchasing a probiotic for your infant, be sure it contains the two different strains, bifidobaceria and lactobacalli, as they are the two most essential bacteria for our health. Most natural health stores carry probiotic drops specifically formulated for infants.

Supplementing your infant's diet with essential fatty acids (EFA's) can be very beneficial to their health and development. Although exclusively breastfed and formula-fed infants get a significant amount of EFA's from their milk, supplementing an infant over the age of 6 months is highly beneficial as these infants are beginning to consume solid foods and less breast milk or formula. EFA supplementation can come from either fish or plants, depending on your preference, as both are beneficial.

Constipation

Constipation is uncomfortable for everyone, especially those little guys who can't voice out their frustration with more than a cry when their tummies aren't feeling well.

Constipation is common and can happen to children as young as 6 months, when solid foods are usually introduced, as well as to older children. The extremity can vary from child to child. Infants who are just starting on solid foods usually develop constipation at some point if the foods they are consuming are not being digested and breaking down properly in order to easily pass through the body in the form of stool. Constipation is rare among infants younger than 6 months of age, especially breastfed babies, but it is possible and can cause a great deal of discomfort.

Note that bowel movements are different between infants, just like adults. Some will have bowel movements three times a day, while others will only have one bowel movement a week, and to them, this may be completely normal. But if all of a sudden those scheduled bowel movements go off track and you are witnessing a cranky child who usually has a good three bowel movements a day not have a single one in a week, you are most likely dealing with a constipated baby.

Symptoms

Keep an eye out for these symptoms of constipation, and monitor your child's bowel movements if you suspect that they may be constipated:

1. Your baby is crying and miserable and has discomfort and pain while trying to pass a stool.

2. Your baby has fewer than three bowel movements a week unless, as mentioned above, this is the norm for your child.

3. Your baby has hard, pellet-like stools that are difficult to push out.

4. Your baby has a hard, bloated belly. Some babies have a naturally bloated belly, so do a feel test with your fingers and lightly press down on your baby's belly. If it feels as though it's very firm and not pressing down much, this may very well be a sign that your baby is backed up.

5. Your baby has a lack of appetite. If your baby has not passed any stool recently, which is basically all of his/her food digested since the last bowel movement, his/her appetite may decrease as there is just not a lot of room left for food if the digested food has not made its way out.

Causes

Formula feeding moms, your baby does have a higher risk of becoming constipated, as formula is usually harder to digest than mother's milk. There is really nothing you can do to prevent this if you are unable or choose not to breastfeed. You may find that your baby's stools are a lot more firm and bulky than a breastfed baby's stools, which are usually soft.

The introduction of solid foods is another common way that infants become constipated. When they begin eating a new food that is not milk, it may take some time for their bodies to learn to manage digesting these new foods. Ensure your infant's first foods are full of fibre and water. Foods such as pureed organic fruits and vegetables are perfect sources of high fibre and water.

Dehydration can often cause constipation in infants as well as in younger children, as water is needed to help break down food particles and lubricate so that food is easily passed from the body. If your infant is not drinking as much milk as usual due to an illness or teething, which may suppress appetite, this can leave him/her dehydrated. If this is the case, offer him/her smaller, more frequent feedings throughout the day. Infants who are consuming solids, may also not be taking enough liquid in-between their meals. Be sure to always have fresh water or milk available, and offer it to them often. Giving your infant enough fluids to prevent him/her from getting dehydrated will help prevent and treat constipation in most cases.

On some rare occasions, a specific medicine or supplement that your infant has been taking may cause temporary constipation. In this case, the best way to get relief is to keep your baby hydrated and wait until the medication has been stopped. Hopefully by then his/her bowel movements will have returned to normal.

How to treat constipation

The best way to treat constipation is to prevent it from happening. Unfortunately, once it has happened it may take a few days to get the bowels properly functioning again and bowel movements to start occurring.

Some doctors may offer a gentle laxative for baby, but I highly suggest not giving your baby any kind of medicinal laxative at that age. When the body begins taking in laxatives to get the colon moving again, it may begin to rely on this method for having bowel movements. While it may provide immediate relief in most cases, once the laxatives are no longer being used, the colon may become sluggish again and the constipation may return.

The best way to defeat constipation is to do so in a natural fashion. Here are some excellent natural remedies you can try at home before consulting a doctor. If the constipation appears to be getting worse or bowel movements have not been present for over a week, medical advice and a gentle laxative may be needed temporarily.

1. Bicycle legs! Lay your baby gently on his/her back and bring his/her knees up to his/her belly, one after another, in a rotating motion like how your legs would work while riding a bicycle. Start doing this movement for about 1 minute, then switch to both legs at the same time being brought up to the belly and back down. Repeat this for another minute. This technique works incredibly well, especially to help remove gas locked up in a baby's intestines, as the gentle pressure helps move gas and food along the colon.

2. Formula switch up: If you are a mother who is bottle-feeding with formula, you may want to consider trying a different brand or a different form of formula. If your baby is drinking a traditional dairy-based formula, it could be that your baby is sensitive to dairy, or dairy is just too difficult for your baby to digest at this stage in life. Try opting for a goat milk-based formula. Although this may be harder to find and can be more expensive, it is far more gentle on the digestive system than cow's milk as it contains less lactose (the sugar found in cow's milk). I would not recommend soy as covered previously, as soy can cause more problems than just constipation. If goat's milk is not an option, try switching to an organic formula if not already using one or to a different brand name that might have slightly different ingredients.

3. If your baby is at the stage of eating solids, lots of fresh water and pure, organic prune juice may help loosen things up! Choose high fibre foods such as apples, apricots, pears, prunes, plums, and lots of vegetables such as yams and green beans. If your child is older and has begun eating grains, a high-fibre hot cereal with lots of water may help get things moving. Again, it is important to not allow your child to drink liquids during meals, but rather in-between, as the digestive acids used to break down foods in the stomach become diluted, and we want to make digestion as strong as possible during this time.

4. Belly rubs! Your baby and you will love these. Lay baby gently down on a soft blanket or your bed and use some natural lotion or oil, such as coconut or olive. (I love mixing some lovely lavender essential oil in with my lotions and oils, as it leaves a soft scent and is great for calming baby.) Start by making small to big, clockwise motions with your three middle fingers closed together, working your way all around your baby's tummy. Begin making the same motion circles going the opposite way, and repeat for a couple of minutes. Just like the bicycle legs, this gentle rubbing of the stomach helps to activate the colon and pass the stool along.

Constipation occurs naturally from time to time and it isn't something to worry about, as there are many natural ways to treat this problem when it happens. Unfortunately, sometimes it isn't easy on baby or on the parents, but do your best to comfort your little one and this phase will soon come to pass. I recommend noting your child's bowel movements on the calendar or in a notebook so you can be completely aware of any sudden changes that may be the beginning of constipation.

Chapter 12
Food Allergies

Hidden food allergies!

A scary but normal and easily fixable situation is when your infant first comes in contact with a food allergen. This can easily happen at any age, but is commonly seen when infants are being introduced to solids.

You may in fact assume that just because your child experiences discomfort after eating a certain food, he or she is having an allergic reaction. However, it may in fact be a food sensitivity, which is more common than the typical allergy. Keep an eye out when introducing new foods to baby and learn to spot the difference between food induced sensitivities and actual allergies.

A food allergy usually causes an immediate immune system reaction, such as air passages being closed, a sudden breakout of hives, or numbing and tingling of the lips, tongue or face. It can even be life-threatening such as with anaphylaxis, which can cause breathing problems and dangerously low blood pressure. Even the smallest amount of an offending food that your body considers an allergen can cause a severe and immediate reaction. These foods need to be completely avoided until being assessed by a doctor or naturopath, as they may be safe for re-introduction later. More allergic reaction symptoms to keep an eye out for are digestive problems such as diarrhea, nausea, and vomiting.

Food sensitive are quite different. They are usually less serious and limited to digestive system problems. Unlike food allergens, food sensitivity symptoms usually come on gradually. If your child does consume a food that he or she may be sensitive to, they display mild to moderate symptoms such as constipation, diarrhea, gas, bloating, skin problems (eczema or diaper rash), and colic.

The most common causes of food sensitivities in infants are:
1. Celiac disease: This usually develops in infants but can easily develop later in adulthood. Some cases of celiac disease are more severe than others as it does to an extent involve the

immune system and can even be life-threatening. Celiac disease usually triggers symptoms in the gastrointestinal system and is brought on by the consumption of eating gluten, a protein found in wheat and other non-gluten-free grains.

2. Absence or lack of a specific enzyme needed to digest a certain food completely: The most common case of enzyme deficiency responsible for causing food intolerance is lactase. Those lacking this enzyme are usually lactose intolerant, as their body cannot digest the lactose (sugar) in the dairy milk.

3. Sensitivities to food additives: This can easily be a main trigger for infants who consume a lot of processed foods such as hot dogs, candy, cookies, and crackers. To avoid any food additives, feed your children whole, organic, and unprocessed foods. There are many healthy alternatives to "baby snacks" which don't contain any food additives and are completely natural.

Allergy elimination diet

The allergy elimination diet has been a popular and worldwide meal plan that avoids the trigger food to which a person may be sensitive. It is fairly simple, but does restrict a variety of foods that are considered to be a "high allergen". Avoid these foods until later in your infant's life (usually around a year is a good time to start introduction of these foods), or eliminate one of these foods a week until the food sensitivity has been pointed out. Use this method if your infant has been regularly eating these foods, and you've noticed any of the above symptoms of a food allergy or sensitivity.

The most common trigger foods for allergies and sensitivities are:
- Citrus fruits such as oranges, lemons, limes, and grapefruit
- Tomatoes, eggplant, potatoes (sweet potato and yams are ok)
- All gluten containing products including corn
- All soy containing products, including organic
- All nuts and seeds including milks (use rice or gluten-free oat milk as a substitute)
- All fish including shellfish
- Pork
- All dairy products, including organic
- Processed foods of any kind
- Sugar, not including fruit

There is quite a variety of food to be removed while participating in the allergy elimination diet, but it is only temporary, and in many cases, most of these food items can be safely returned to your child's diet.

Once all of these products have been taken out of your baby's diet for at least a week (some prefer even two weeks), you may start adding in one of the restricted foods a week into your baby's diet. During this time it is very crucial that you take note of any allergen symptoms you notice once a certain food has been re introduced. Remember, just one food per week, as multiple allergen foods can throw off which food is giving which symptom. Once you notice a symptom being displayed by your child that is out of the ordinary, I suggest removing that specific item from their diet. Many alternative foods are available.

Continue on until you've reached every food on the list, removing any food that triggered an allergen symptom. Although your child may have a reaction to that specific food in his or her life right now, it may not reoccur once the child is older. It is recommend those foods be reintroduced in another allergy elimination diet after the age of one.

Chapter 13
My Not-so-little Baby: Nutrition for the Growing Toddler and Child

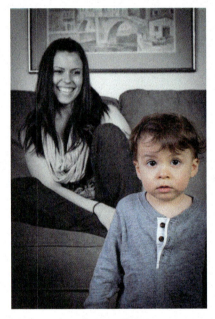

You come first photography

Quality over quantity

As your infant becomes a toddler and continues to grow, their nutritional values stand the same, just in larger amounts. Your child will go through many growth spurts, and as parents, it is your job to provide the highest quality nutrients to support that growing body! Your baby has now said good-bye to the strained, blended, and pureed forms of food and hello to the crunchy, bulky, textured, I-can-eat-with-my-fingers-and-fork type of foods. This is great because your child can now eat practically anything that you eat, making your job much easier!

Although your toddler has seemed to grow at an enormous rate since birth, it will now slow down to about 3.5 inches a year. During this time, you will notice a slight increase in appetite. This is only natural, as your toddler becomes larger and more active. Don't worry about how many calories he or she is taking in, but focus more on the nutrient content. Quality over quantity! If your child is constantly eating, and you're worried that you are overfeeding him, don't be.

Your child at his/her age, knows exactly how to listen to his/her body – unlike adults who can eat way pass the "full" point and become over-satiated. Children know exactly when they are full and when to stop. Just because your toddler has a much bigger appetite does not increase the chances of that child becoming obese or overweight. It could simply be that his/her energy output is much higher than some other children who eat much less. As long as you are focusing on a whole-foods diet, you will not have to worry about your child gaining excess weight.

The same goes for a child who eats very small portions compared to other children. However, if your child is measuring smaller than average and is not improving in the growth category over the year, you may want to have your child seen regularly by a doctor to ensure there is not a more serious medical concern, rather than your child simply not being hungry.

Up it to gain it

If your child does not seem to be gaining weight at the recommended pace for his/her age, you will need to compensate by adding extra calories and more EFA's to his/her meals. It can be difficult if your child refuses to eat, but there are ways to get those extra calories in when your child least expects it.

You can increase your child's calorie intake by:

1. Supplementing his/her diet with more breast milk or formula feedings. If your child is no longer nursing or receiving formula, supplementing his/her diet with whole organic milk or goat's milk will help increase calorie intake as it has a very high fat content.

2. Adding more healthy fats like avocado, olive or coconut oil, or organic butter to their meals.

3. Adding flax seed oil to their water or other beverages, including breast milk or formula, as it will increase fat content without necessarily giving them more bulky foods.

4. Offering more snacks and meals more frequently throughout the day.

If your child is simply smaller than average, but is still increasing in growth, I wouldn't worry too much and not force any more food than he/she can handle on the plate. Keep snacks around for easy access that your child can pick at when hungry. But remember, it may just be that your little one has a smaller appetite. If he or she is healthy and your doctor does not have any concerns, don't push it. Their appetite will eventually increase over time.

Let's get fat: The benefits of essential fatty acids (EFA'S)

As your baby is consuming less breast milk or formula, his/her essential fatty acid levels may be slowly decreasing, which we want to prevent.

Essential fatty acids are extremely important in your child's diet, especially during the first few years after birth, as this is when the brain is growing and developing rapidly. EFA's are fatty acids that humans must consume through diet, as our bodies cannot synthesize them, and they are essential for good health, as mentioned in our earlier chapters about healthy eating for expecting mothers.

Many babies are actually deficient in the recommended amount of EFA's to maintain a healthy brain. These fats are responsible for building cells (especially brain cells, as our brains are made mostly of fat), regulating the nervous system, strengthening the cardiovascular system while building up a strong immune system. They also allow for the absorption of fat-soluble vitamins.

From age 1 to 3 your child should be obtaining 0.7 grams of omega 3 fatty acids daily. By adding some avocado to their smoothies and coconut or extra virgin olive oil to their vegetable dishes, you will never have to be concerned that your baby is not getting enough. Other great sources are wild salmon, flax seed oil, and organic butter, which can be easily mixed into any food and does not have much of a taste. Having the appropriate amount of EFA's in your child's diet will ensure proper brain function, growth, and development.

If you are concerned that your child is not consuming adequate amounts of essential fatty acids, supplements with a natural fish oil or plant-based EFA's is an option.

The RDA

The recommended dietary allowance or RDA is the average daily dietary intake level that is sufficient to meet the nutrition requirements of healthy individuals, depending on age and gender.

These are the RDA's for the top essential vitamins recommended for ultimate health.

RDA for children 1 to 13 years of age:

1. Vitamin A: 300 to 600 micrograms
2. Vitamin C: 15 to 45 Mg
3. Vitamin D: 15 micrograms
4. Vitamin E: 6 to 11 mg

By feeding your child a well-balanced, whole-foods diet with lots of variety, you will have no problem meeting or exceeding the recommended dosage of the daily requirements.

Excellent sources of vitamin A include:
- Sweet potatoes
- Carrots
- Spinach
- Dark leafy greens (kale, mustard greens, collard greens, Swiss chard)
- Winter squash

Excellent sources of vitamin C include:
- Papaya
- Bell peppers
- Broccoli
- Oranges
- Strawberries

Excellent sources of vitamin D include:
- Sunshine!
- Wild salmon
- Free-range eggs

Excellent sources of vitamin E include:
- Raw Sunflower seeds
- Raw almonds
- Spinach
- Avocado
- Asparagus

Ensure that whenever possible, you choose organic produce, as its vitamin and mineral content are much higher and easier to be absorbed by the body as they are not affected by the use of pesticides and herbicides.

Fussy eaters

Although you may be trying your best to give your child the best nutrition possible, you may just be one of the many unfortunate parents who have a fussy eater in the house. This is perfectly normal and more common than you may think. Who doesn't hate eating veggies when they are two? Do your best to give your child a variety of different foods so that his/her palate can get used to different flavours and textures. Remember, it can take up to ten times of trying the same food for your child to actually like it! So don't give up, just because he/she won't eat it now. Keep trying every day or a few times a week and eventually he/she may come to realize it isn't that bad. Of course you are going to get the occasional food that your child will never put near his/her mouth until they are in their late twenties, but that won't be the situation for every food.

A good tip for parents dealing with fussy eaters is to make food fun or to camouflage those healthy goods in meals they really enjoy. Create a salad bar with a variety of vegetables that allows your child the sense of being independent and where he or she can choose what colourful veggies they want to go on top of their greens. Include options like slivered almonds, dried cranberries, and a couple choices of healthy dressing to top off the salad. The beautiful art and creativity in front of your child might just give him/her the push he/she needs to try something new!

Another great secret for feeding a fussy eater is the camouflage method. Hide those greens and other vegetables in dishes your child already eats on a day-to-day basis. Blend some spinach in your pancake batter by placing all the ingredients in a high-powered blender. When the spinach is cooked, not only will the flavour be completely hidden, but what you get left with is amazingly cool, green-coloured pancakes! What kid wouldn't want to eat that? You can even do the old blending greens and other healthy additives like flax seeds into a smoothie packed with fruit. The green colour will still be there, but the flavour will be covered up with all the sweet, juicy fruit. Allow your child to be part of the culinary experience and get them interested in preparing meals early in life. They will soon realize how amazing food really is with all its unique flavours and colours.

If you still feel that after everything you are doing, progress is just too slow and your child is lacking in certain vitamins and minerals, fear not. Supplementing your child's diet with a high-quality multivitamin will ensure he/she is getting the daily recommended dosage. Supplements should not replace real food, but can assist in giving your child all he or she needs if they are in the stage of fussy eating. It will eventually pass, so stay patient and remember to get creative!

To sum it all up, nutrition for your child is one of the most important aspects for maintaining good health and overall wellness. Nutrition is the key to giving your growing child everything he or she needs to thrive in life and should not be taken lightly.

Feed your child a diet of organic, fresh, whole, natural and unprocessed foods to ensure he/she is getting the highest quality of vitamins and minerals possible for his/her growing mind and body.

By avoiding foods harmful to the body and promoting foods from the earth, your child's learning ability will increase. Catching illnesses will be limited as his/her immune systems will be very strong to fight off germs, and their overall mood will be much more positive. Your child will be vibrant and thriving when on a whole-foods diet!

Chapter 14
Veggie Baby

No meat, no problem

In today's society we see more and more people turning away from carnivore diets and focusing more on plant-based diets. As more research is being done, it's being shown that adopting a high plant-based diet is very healthy for humans. Even if we are eating meat, reducing the amounts and eating more plant-based food may save us from a lot of food-related illness such as obesity, diabetes, and heart attacks.

So what about children who are adopting a plant-based diet or have simply been brought up that way from birth due to their parents' decisions or beliefs? Can they be just as healthy with no meat in their diet? How about vegan children? Will they be just as healthy with no meat, dairy, eggs, or any animal byproducts in their diet? The answer is: OF COURSE!

We don't necessarily need meat or other animal products in our lives to be healthy. We can easily survive on a 100 percent plant-based diet, as long as we are eating a balance of the right foods and a rotating between foods to ensure we are getting all the nutrients we need from plants.

Many mothers often ask me where children who live off of plant-based diets get their protein from, if they get enough, and if they will be deficient and lack growth without having animal flesh in their diet. I tell them all the same thing. No matter which way of eating we practise, the same rules apply: whole foods, organic, fresh, balanced, and variation. By following those 5 simple guidelines, anyone can sustain health, even if they don't include a food group in their diet.

What is vegetarian?

A vegetarian is an individual who does not include meat in his/her diet. Some may include dairy, eggs, and fish. This way of eating can very healthy, but at the same time, it can be just as unhealthy as someone who consumes meat. When people hear the word "vegetarian", they assume that person must practise a healthy way of eating with tons of vegetables, hence the name. But in a lot of cases, many vegetarians get the majority of their caloric intake from unhealthy sources of food such as full-fat cheese, milk and yogurt, white bread, rice and pasta, and too many eggs. There are also the junk foods such as chips, pop, cookies, and ice cream. There are many unhealthy food choices that do not include meats, so if you do plan on raising your child as a vegetarian, you must focus on real, whole foods and away from processed junk food.

At the same time, there are many vegetarians who do practise a well balanced diet. These individuals focus on plenty of whole grains, organic eggs, wild caught fish (for those who choose to include it), low-fat organic dairy, and an abundance of fresh fruit and vegetables.

You want your vegetarian child to thrive on these healthy foods to ensure he/she is obtaining all the essential nutrients for his/her growing body. Supplements are not usually needed or recommended when eating a healthy vegetarian diet because you can obtain the nutrients from meat by consuming eggs and fish. A multivitamin is always suggested as a back-up for a lack of one or more nutrients.

What is a vegan?

A vegan is an individual who follows a much stricter version of a vegetarian diet. Vegans do not include ANY animal products in their diet including, eggs, fish, milk, butter, or gelatin. Because these ingredients are contained in so many processed foods in our markets, it can make vegan grocery shopping a little more complicated, as it is important to read the ingredients for many items. A vegan diet is essentially more healthy than a traditional vegetarian diet as it does not allow for all the high-fat dairy products such as cheese and ice cream. However, there is still vegan junk food, such as baked goods, pastas, candy, chocolate, and artificial meats which contain high amounts of fat and sodium.

Getting enough: Balance is key

A vegan diet is also one that needs extra consideration when making sure the diet is well balanced. Variation in this diet is also quite important as there are a few essential nutrients you cannot obtain from this diet. Eating a variety of different vegan foods will ensure you are getting enough nutrients to keep your body as healthy as possible. This is especially important when raising vegan children, as many vegan children are deficient in certain nutrients due to a lack of certain foods.

Vitamin B12 and vitamin D are the two most important ones that must be supplemented in a vegan diet, as one can only obtain them from animal products. Many vegans are deficient in vitamin B12 and sometimes may not realize it. When not getting the recommended dosage of this B vitamin, you may experience symptoms of fatigue, confusion or a change in mental state, depression, and/or a loss of balance. A B12 deficiency in a child can be extremely dangerous, and supplements are needed to prevent this. Nutritional yeast, which is the only plant-based food that has a high level of Vitamin B12, can be added to meals to increase the daily dosage.

Vitamin D supplements, just like with infants, can be given orally at a 400 IU dosage twice a day. Vitamin D also helps to ensure that the body is absorbing and retaining the minerals calcium and phosphorus. These two minerals are crucial for bone development and strength.

As long as your child is being supplemented with B12 and vitamin D when following a vegan diet, there is no need to question if they are deficient. Ensure your child is consuming a balance of proteins, healthy fats, and complex carbohydrates to get the maximum benefits of being vegan.

The protein myth around veganism has been greatly busted over the years. Society used to constantly taunt vegans for not getting enough protein in their diet and for being small and weak. This is not the case. There are many sources of vegan proteins that can fulfill the recommended amount needed to maintain muscle mass. The only difference between vegan protein and animal protein is that a lot of vegan proteins are not complete proteins, while animal proteins are. A complete protein is one that contains all nine of the essential amino acids. Amino acids are the building blocks of the body and are responsible for muscle building and repair, controlling the body's insulin, and maintaining healthy hair, skin, and nails.

The best way to ensure your child is getting all the essential amino acids in his/her diet with the absence of meat is to combine grains and legumes in the diet. By combining grains such as oats, millet, brown rice, or buckwheat with legumes like chickpeas, lentils, or navy beans, you are sure to get all of the essential amino acids.

Balance your child's diet with proper sized portions of these different combos throughout the day. They don't even have to be in the same meal, as long as whole grains and legumes are being consumed daily. Quinoa, a seed, but commonly known as an ancient super-food grain, contains all of the essential amino acids, and is one of the only plant-based foods that is considered to be a complete protein!

Calcium, another nutrient that some individuals may be lacking when consuming a vegan diet because of the avoidance of dairy, can easily be obtained by consuming a good portion of leafy greens, such as kale, Swiss chard, and collard greens. Spinach is another excellent source of calcium, but due to it being moderately high in oxalates, which can decrease calcium absorption, it should be gently steamed or sautéed.

If you find greens aren't really your forte, sesame seeds, which contain the highest source of calcium, can be added to your diet simply by adding a tablespoon on top of your salads or in smoothies, or by making a sesame bar with raw honey. Other great sources are raw hazelnuts, almonds, Brazil nuts, and pumpkin and sunflower seeds. A high quality calcium supplement can be taken once a day if needed.

Since your child is not consuming any animal products, and plants are naturally low in fat, adding some essential fat into your child's diet will prevent EFA deficiency, as mentioned previously. EFA's are very important to growing children, especially for brain development. Fat is higher in calories than carbohydrates and protein, therefore it must be eaten in moderation and not overdone. A small serving of added healthy fats with each meal is enough to provide the recommended daily serving.

All in all, children who eat a whole, plant-based diet receive the same nutrients as those who eat meat. Although vegan diets may take a little more time and energy to plan, they eventually become second nature, and it can be very simple to obtain all the essential nutrients. Because plant-based diets are so high in fibre, they are highly recommended for children struggling with constipation.

Hydration for your growing child

Water is the most essential element for all living beings. Childhood hydration is just as important as infant hydration. Keeping your children hydrated is crucial and goes hand in hand when feeding them a nutritious diet! Water is needed to fuel your children's growth, play, and life! Pure, filtered water should be the focus of hydration when it comes to your little one; not milk, not apple juice, but water! It fills those little bodies with goodness and flushes out all the bad stuff such as toxic build-up that might have accumulated from the air, food, and other environmental factors.

As difficult as it can be to get adults to drink enough water, getting your child to drink lots of water may be the impossible. Keeping a water bottle in arms' reach from your infant whenever possible is a great way for them to begin hydrating themselves without even knowing it! They will automatically reach for the bottle and drink numerous times while playing. Try finding a water bottle or sippy cup that has some fun characters illustrated on the sides that get your child's attention to help increase the amount of water consumed.

I highly recommend adding some natural water flavours to further entice your child to drink more water. Slicing some organic strawberries and cucumber and infusing a jug of filtered water overnight will allow for a healthy and hydrating treat the next morning. Store the jug in your fridge for the day to keep it fresh, and you'll be amazed to see the water level go down as your child gulps it.

Fresh juices are another great way to get your child hydrated. Although they should not replace water, they are a nice and nutritious treat to have. Fresh fruit and vegetable juices contain a large amount of nutrients as well as water content from the fruits and vegetables. It also tastes really good, and the colours are stunning!

I allow my little one to sip on natural coconut water throughout the day. Its low amount of sugar can help fuel your little one's daily activities without the side effects of a sugar crash. It's another great tasting, slightly sweet beverage with many health benefits that your child will be sure to love!

As your child grows and learns the benefits of good nutrition, he/she will continue practising those values as they grow into healthy teenagers and through to adulthood. Setting up a child with all the tools to a healthy diet early in life will be setting them up for a lifetime of health and wellness. And remember parents: Monkey see, monkey do. So you as parents are responsible for practising good eating habits in front of your little one. They will watch you, learn from you, and live by your knowledge, so let us gear up and be the greatest role models to our children as possible.

Chapter 15
Eating for Mental Health

During my years of gaining experience in a holistic nutrition practice, I focused a lot of my studies around children with mental disorders such as autism and ADHD. After doing about a year of research on how diet can potentially affect these disorders, I decided to take my research, and the research and knowledge of others, to the next level.

I enrolled in a part-time career working with autistic and ADHD children as a behavioural therapist assistant. Through this career, which lasted about a year, I was given a wonderful opportunity by the parents of these children to test my research. I began implementing diets that targeted their disorders to see if certain foods acted as triggers that made their situation better or worse. I found that the research around autism and ADHD when correlating it with food seemed to be very accurate.

All of the foods found in each child's diet were quite similar, and when removed, had the same effect on each child with the same level of effectiveness. I tried this specific diet with about five different children from different families, and in my eyes, it had a major positive effect on their lifestyle.

What is autism?

Autism, also known as autism spectrum disorder, as the dictionary states, is a mental condition present from early childhood. The condition is distinguished by difficulty in communication and social interactions with others.

What is ADHD?

ADHD, also known as attention deficit hyperactivity disorder, is a condition that commonly affects children and young adults. It can easily continue through to adulthood without proper treatment. Children diagnosed with this disorder usually display symptoms of hyperactivity, anxiety, and over excitability and have trouble focusing on certain tasks. ADHD can impair a child's ability to function and be accepted socially and academically.

Autism and ADHD have been shown to be closely linked in many children, making life more challenging for the child and the parent. Implementing a certain diet that is targeted for children with this disorder may help reduce the signs of autism and ADHD. Although this diet may not work for every child, and its success depends on the severity of the disorder, several parents who have implemented a specific diet have reported that it did in fact improve their child's mental state.

The GFCF diet

The GFCF diet is simply one with no gluten (the protein that is found in wheat and many other grains) and casein (a protein present in all dairy products). Although there has been very little research done on the GFCF diet for children with autism and ADHD, I highly recommend that parents try it with their children, as many recommend it.

Some parents believe that their children are allergic or sensitive to these two proteins, so removing them reduces symptoms of anxiety, confusion, and hyperactivity. Research by Dr. Harumi Jyonouchi has shown that 91% of people with autism who were put on a strict, gluten-free, casein-free, sugar-free diet improved. Jyonouchi's research papers say that ASD children have an aberrant immune response to the dietary proteins found in gluten, casein, and soy.

Gluten and casein are not the only culprits I have found when working with children with this disorder. Sugar also has negative effects on these children's mental states. Children today are still getting 15% more sugar than the recommended daily percentage. With such a large dosage of these sugars, children are experiencing more behavioural and learning difficulties, as well as much shorter attention spans; behaviors that are already present in autistic and ADHD kids.

Not all sugars are bad, and I don't recommend restricting all of them, especially the natural sugars found in fruit. Fruit juice, however, is not recommended. It is concentrated sugar and in high amounts can negatively affect the nervous system as much as white sugar. If you are giving your child juice, I would recommend diluting it with water, or severely cutting back to half a cup per day. However, it is best to completely avoid it.

Sugar also causes highs, which eventually lead to a sugar crash a few hours after the sugar was ingested. Some children can be more sensitive than others, but the results are often very similar.

When a crash happens, it leaves the individual feeling sluggish and drained and with low blood sugar, which can lead to abnormal behaviour.

Feed your child a whole-foods diet and limit sugar consumption with no products containing gluten and casein. At first this may be a challenge, especially getting your children used to the taste of many gluten- and casein-free alternatives. But with time and creativeness, they will become used to it. I find that many of the gluten- and dairy-free products on the shelves of grocery stores are loaded with too much sugar and artificial ingredients, with the exceptions of organic options from health stores. However, even these can contain too much natural sugar.

I recommend purchasing a couple gluten-free/dairy-free cookbooks or downloading some recipes from the Internet. That way, if a recipe calls for sugar, you can replace it using a lower sugar substitute such as mashed banana, applesauce, or stevia. Homemade baking is a better option as it's fresh, and you know exactly what ingredients are being added.

Keep track of your child's progress and stay as strict as possible with the guidelines. Slip-ups can result in a large step backwards for your child's treatment. A food log is highly recommended as you can easily log your child's meals and beverages and mark any improvements you see along the way. It's very motivating to see positive changes in your child's behaviour.

Chapter 16
Recipes and Meal Plan

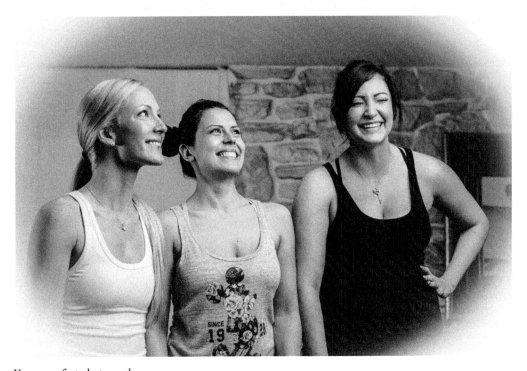

You come first photography

Welcome to my recipe section! All of my recipes have been taste-tested by moms and are filled with nutritious, whole foods! These recipes are appropriate for preconception, pregnancy, postpartum, and the whole family. I have provided a sample 7-day meal plan to help you jump-start your journey to a healthy you and happy baby! The meal plan consists of three main meals, one afternoon snack, and a dessert!

7-Day sample meal plan

Day one
Upon rising and prior to breakfast, sip a warm cup of purified water with a squeeze of fresh lemon. Take one high-quality prenatal or multivitamin with one glass of purified water. You may also have a cup of herbal tea with stevia.

Breakfast:
Little big green smoothie (see recipe)

Snack:
Fresh organic fruit
1 cup of plain or fruit flavoured organic coconut or almond yogurt

Lunch:
1 warmed gluten-free pita or wrap, stuffed with organic goat cheese, hummus, bell pepper, red onion, and sliced avocado.
Enjoy with a side garden salad topped with apple cider or balsamic vinegar.

Dinner:
Mexican quinoa salad (see recipe)

Dessert:
2 squares of organic, dairy-free dark chocolate (at least 70% cocoa)

Day two
Upon rising and prior to breakfast, sip a warm cup of purified water with a squeeze of fresh lemon. Take one high quality prenatal or multivitamin with one glass of purified water. You may also have a cup of herbal tea with stevia.

Breakfast:
Greens in my eggs. Hold the ham! (see recipe)

Snack:
Protein shake. Mix 1 to 2 scoops of a non-soy-based vegan protein powder (see protein powder recommendations) with 1 cup of unsweetened non-dairy milk, ½ banana, 1 cup of kale, and 1 cup of ice in a high-powered blender. Blend until smooth. Serve immediately.

Dinner:
Grilled, free-range chicken breast topped with Mama's Salsa (see recipe), served with 3 baby-baked potatoes and steamed asparagus.

Dessert:
Avocado chocolate pudding (see recipe)

Day three
Upon rising and prior to breakfast, sip a warm cup of purified water with a squeeze of fresh lemon. Take one high quality prenatal or multivitamin with one glass of purified water. You may also have a cup of herbal tea with stevia.

Breakfast:
1 cup of cooked, rolled, or steel-cut oats topped with organic, mixed berries, cinnamon, slivered almonds, and warm coconut milk. Sweeten with stevia.
(For an added benefit, add a greens supplement such as Genuine Health's Greens+. It contains an abundant amount of super foods and phytonutrients.)

Snack:
Gluten-free crackers and fresh vegetable sticks served with hummus.

Lunch:
A large green salad, loaded with fresh chopped vegetables and herbs, topped with 1 cup of chickpeas or chopped, free-range chicken breast.
Dressing: 1 tbsp of organic flax seed oil and 1 tbsp of apple cider or balsamic vinegar.

Dinner:
Vegetarian gluten-free/dairy-free lasagna (see recipe)

Dessert:
½ cup of coconut or rice milk ice cream or try my monkey ice cream (see recipe)

Day four
Upon rising and prior to breakfast, sip a warm cup of purified water with a squeeze of fresh lemon. Take one high quality prenatal or multivitamin with one glass of purified water. You may also have a cup of herbal tea with stevia.

Breakfast:
Mexican scramble burrito (see recipe)

Snack:
Fruit and yogurt parfait
In a bowl or cup, place a layer of fresh berries at the bottom, top with 1 scoop of almond or coconut yogurt, then sprinkle about 1 tbsp of raw oats

or organic granola on top. Repeat steps, creating two more layers. Top with more fresh berries and drizzle with raw honey or brown rice syrup.

Lunch:
1 to 2 slices of gluten-free or sprouted grain bread, toasted, topped with sliced organic tomato, ½ avocado, sea salt, and pepper, and then drizzled with fresh lime juice. (For a spicier version, add a little sprinkle of cayenne pepper on top!)

Dinner:
Vegetarian cabbage rolls

Dessert:
1 raw cocoa truffle ball (see recipe) or 3 large strawberries dipped in 1 tbsp of melted dairy-free, organic dark chocolate.

Day five
Upon rising and prior to breakfast, sip a warm cup of purified water with a squeeze of fresh lemon. Take one high quality prenatal or multivitamin with one glass of purified water. You may also have a cup of herbal tea with stevia.

Breakfast:
Fresh fruit bowl topped with crumbled walnuts, slivered almonds, and chia seeds and drizzled with raw honey or brown rice syrup

Snack:
Gluten-free crackers or gluten-free pita bread and raw veggie sticks dipped in guacamole.

Lunch:
Mama's Tangy Chili (see recipe)

Dinner:
Baked wild salmon, topped with lemon juice and fresh dill. Served with 1 cup of quinoa or brown rice and steamed broccoli tossed in coconut oil.

Dessert:
Handful of organic, dried apples or apricots

Day six
Upon rising and prior to breakfast, sip a warm cup of purified water with a squeeze of fresh lemon. Take one high quality prenatal or multivitamin with one glass of purified water. You may also have a cup of herbal tea with stevia.

Breakfast:
Gluten-free apple spice pancakes (see recipe)

Snack:
1 organic apple, sliced into rings, topped with natural almond butter and raisins

Lunch:
Tempeh Asian Stir-fry (see recipe)

Dinner:
Quinoa and black bean stuffed peppers (see recipe)

Dessert:
Frozen banana half dipped in organic, dairy-free dark chocolate and chopped pecans. (Cut 1 banana in half, place in freezer overnight. Melt 1 tbsp of organic, dairy-free dark chocolate and dip the banana halfway until coated with the chocolate. Quickly, before the chocolate hardens, roll it in the chopped pecans and place in freezer to harden chocolate, about 5 minutes.)

Day seven

Upon rising and prior to breakfast, sip a warm cup of purified water with a squeeze of fresh lemon. Take one high quality prenatal or multivitamin with one glass of purified water. You may also have a cup of herbal tea with stevia.

Breakfast:
Gluten-free waffles, topped with sliced peaches, ground flax seed, dried unsweetened coconut, and then drizzled with pure, organic maple syrup.

Snack:
1 Nature's Mama Granola Bar (see recipe)

Lunch:
Salad in a jar (see recipe)

Dinner:
Organic roast beef, topped with homemade gravy (see recipe), served with cauliflower mash (see recipe) and garlic roasted carrots (see recipe)

Dessert:
½ cup of cinnamon rice pudding (see recipe)

Family recipes

Smoothies and Juices and Bevies

Instructions:

For smoothie, place all ingredients in a high-speed blender for 90 seconds until smooth.

For juice, place ingredients one at a time in the juicer.

Drink immediately for better health benefits.

For other beverages, follow instructions below recipe.

The Little Green Smoothie

½ banana
½ pear
1 lemon wedge (peeled and seeded)
1 large handful of organic spinach or kale
1 cup of coconut water or purified water
1 cup of ice
Stevia to taste

Protein Punch Smoothie

1 scoop of dairy, soy-free, organic protein powder
1 banana
1 cup of frozen strawberries
1 tbsp of bee pollen
2 large handfuls of organic spinach
Stevia to taste
1 cup of unsweetened almond, rice, or coconut milk
4 ice cubes

Rouge Bleu Juice

2 peeled red beets
1 red apple, cored and seeded
2 large carrots

1 cup blueberries

Blueberry Almond Milk

1 cup of almonds (soak almonds overnight)
1 cup of fresh or frozen organic blueberries
3.5 cups of water
2 pitted dates (soak dates overnight)
1 tsp of pure vanilla extract
Few drops of stevia (add more for sweeter tasting milk)
Pinch of sea salt
Once your dates and almonds have been soaked and are soft and tender, add all your ingredients into a high-speed blender.
Blend for a couple of minutes until there are no large chunks.
Using a nut milk bag or cheesecloth, over a large bowl, strain the almond milk through the mesh and squeeze out remaining liquid until nothing but pulp remains in the bag.
Pour almond milk back in the blender and strain once again.
Pour the filtered almond milk in a glass jar or container and refrigerate. Will keep fresh up to 3 to 4 days in the fridge.
Discard the leftover almond pulp or freeze to use in future recipes.
* For vanilla almond milk, omit the blueberries*

French Vanilla Hemp Milk

½ cup organic, shelled hemp hearts
2 dates (soaked overnight)
1 to 2 tsp of pure vanilla extract
Drops of stevia or 1 tbsp of maple syrup (add more for a sweeter tasting milk)
Pinch of sea salt
Place all ingredients into a high-speed blender for about 1 minute, until there are no noticeable chunks.
Using a nut milk bag or cheesecloth, place over a large bowl and strain the hemp milk through the mesh and squeeze out remaining liquid.
Place hemp milk back into blender and strain once again.
Pour the filtered hemp milk into a glass jar or container and refrigerate. Will keep fresh up to 4 days in the fridge.
Discard the left over almond pulp or freeze to use in future recipes

Eggless Egg Nog

4 to 5 cups of homemade vanilla almond or hemp milk (see recipe)
1 tsp of cinnamon
1 tsp of nutmeg

Place ingredients in a high-speed blender and blend for 30 seconds.
Pour into fancy glasses and top with a sprinkle of cinnamon.
Add a few cubes of ice to the blender for a frothy, festive smoothie.

Balance Smoothie or Juice (low sugar)

1 green apple, cut and cored
2 celery sticks
1/3 cucumber
1 cup of kale, stems removed
2 cups of spinach
Stevia to sweeten
1 cup of cold water or coconut water (only for smoothie)
Ice cubes (only for smoothie)

Pumpkin Pie Flax Smoothie

1 cup of homemade vanilla almond or hemp milk
½ cup of organic canned pumpkin
1 tbsp of pure maple syrup
½ ripe banana
2 tsp of ground flax seed
½ tsp of nutmeg
½ tsp of cinnamon
½ to 1 scoop of vegan vanilla protein powder
Ice cubes

Avocado Dreamsicle Smoothie

¼ ripe avocado
1 frozen banana
1 orange, peeled
1 cup of coconut milk
1 large handful of spinach or kale

Stevia to sweeten
Ice cubes

Orange Blossom Juice

1 large orange, peeled
1 mandarin orange, peeled
2 large carrots
1 lemon, peeled
½ grapefruit, peeled
Stevia to taste

Gold Immunity

1.5 cups of homemade vanilla almond or hemp milk
½ tsp of organic, powdered turmeric
¼ to ½ tsp of organic, powdered ginger
Pure maple syrup, raw honey, or stevia to sweeten
Pinch of ground black pepper
In a small pot on medium heat, bring milk to a boil then reduce immediately to low heat. Whisk in other ingredients and remove pan from element, allowing the milk to cool slightly. Pour into a mug or teacup and drink immediately.

Like a Virgin Caesar Cocktail

3 tbsp of lime juice
4.5 cups of organic vegetable juice (similar to V8)
3 tbsp of lemon juice
2 tsp of hot sauce
1 to 2 tbsp of vegan Worcestershire sauce
Tsp of celery seed
Sea salt and black pepper to taste
Celery stalks for garnish
Place all ingredients except celery stalk in a high-speed blender for 60 seconds. Pour into tall glasses and garnish with celery sticks

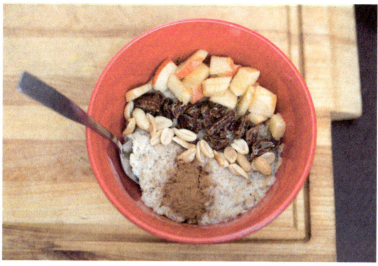

You come first photography

Breakfast

Greens In My eggs. Hold the ham!

2 organic, free-range eggs
1 cup of spinach
¼ green onion, diced
½ large tomato, diced
½ tbsp of coconut oil
1 tbsp of Mama's guacamole or Mama's salsa (see recipe)

Begin by heating coconut oil in a large pan. Add in the vegetables and sauté until tender. While the vegetables are cooking, crack the 4 eggs into a small bowl and scramble with a pinch of sea salt and pepper. Once the vegetables are soft, add the eggs into the pan. Cook the eggs until the top is no longer watery, and flip. Cook other side for 2 more minutes. Spread the guacamole or salsa onto the cooked egg and fold in half. Cut in two with a sharp knife and place on two separate plates. Top each omelette with a sprig of fresh parsley.

Mexican Breakfast Burrito

Serves 4
1 small sweet potato, steamed and cubed
1 cup of cooked black beans
1 large tomato, diced

1 avocado, diced
1 large onion, diced fine
2 tsp of coconut oil
½ cup of Mama's salsa (see recipe)

In a large pan, heat coconut oil on medium heat. Add in onions and sauté until translucent. Add in the sweet potato cubes, tomato, black beans, and avocado, and sauté until the potatoes are slightly crispy. Add in the ½ cup of Mama's salsa, until the mixture is evenly coated. Serve mixture on gluten-free tortillas, wrap, and enjoy!

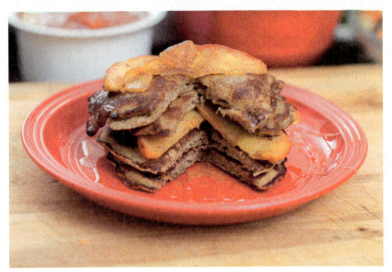

You come first photography

*Apple Spice Pancakes (gluten-free, dairy-free)

Serves 2
1 apple, chopped
½ tsp nutmeg
1 tsp cinnamon
5 drops of liquid stevia or 1 tsp of powered stevia (use more or less for desired sweetness)
1/3 cup brown rice or quinoa flour
¼ cup gluten-free rolled oats
1/3 cup of unsweetened almond, rice, or coconut milk
1 organic egg or egg substitute (if vegan)
1 tsp of pure vanilla extract
½ cup organic applesauce

In a griddle or non-stick pan, on medium heat, use a small amount of virgin coconut oil to evenly coat the surface.

Once oil is hot, sauté the chopped apple, along with the stevia, nutmeg, and cinnamon until the apple is soft.
Once apple mixture is cooked, place half of the mixture in a separate bowl and the other half in a high-speed blender or food processor along with the other ingredients. Blend on high until batter is smooth.
Using the same pan or griddle, coat the surface with another small amount of coconut oil.
Using a ladle or measuring cup, pour ¼ cup of the batter onto the pan and cook both sides until bubbly and slightly golden.
Top the cooked pancakes with other half of apple mixture.
To add a little crunch, sprinkle on some toasted pecans or walnuts

Breakfast Bliss Jar

An easy way to eat on the go, you can even make this overnight and store it in the fridge until the next morning. Busy moms swear by it. No more excuses to why you have to skip breakfast! All you need is a mason jar and these delicious ingredients!
1st layer (bottom): Coconut or organic goats milk yogurt
2nd layer: Fresh blueberries, raspberries, and strawberries
3rd layer: 1 bar of Mama's granola bars (see recipe), crumbled
4th layer: sprinkle of unsweetened, shredded coconut

Main Dishes

Vegetarian Lasagna (gluten-free/dairy-free)

Serves approx. 8
Filling
1 large onion, chopped
2 medium garlic cloves, minced
¼ cup nutritional yeast
4 cups of fresh spinach
½ cup of soy-free, vegan cheese such as Diaya cheese, shredded
1 avocado, peeled and pitted
Lasagna
5 cups of organic marinara sauce or Mama's tomato sauce (see recipe)
12 cooked gluten-free lasagna strips
½ cup of soy-free vegan cheese, shredded
Nutritional yeast and chopped parsley for topping

To prepare the filling:

Preheat the oven to 400 degrees Fahrenheit. In a large saucepan, heat about ¼ cup of water and sauté your onion and garlic until soft. Add in your spinach and stir until spinach is slightly wilted. Do not overcook. In a food processor, add your onion, garlic, and spinach mix. Remove the flesh from the avocado and add it to your food processor along with the nutritional yeast. Pulse until smooth.

Spread a hearty amount of marinara sauce on the bottom of a large glass pan, and then cover with about 4 noodles. Top the noodles with about ½ of the avocado filling. Repeat steps until all the noodles and filling are in the pan. You should have the top layer ending the lasagna. Top the lasagna with the remaining marinara sauce, vegan cheese, nutritional yeast, and parsley. Cover the lasagna with parchment paper or an oven-safe lid. Bake for about 30 minutes or until the cheese is bubbly and brown. Let cool before serving

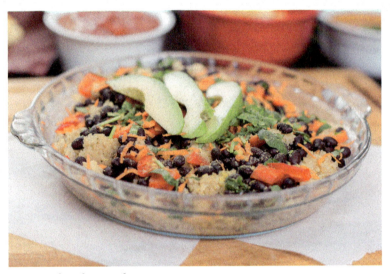

You come first photography

Mexican Couscous Salad

Serves 2

2 cups of cooked couscous (cook in organic vegetable broth for more flavour)

2 cups of cooked black beans (if canned, use organic, drain and rinse)

1 cup of organic corn kernels (steamed fresh or canned)

1 red bell pepper, diced

½ cup finely minced red onion

1 to 2 tbsp of chopped cilantro

½ avocado, diced

1 cup of Mama's salsa (see recipe)

Juice of one lime

Combine all ingredients, except for the cilantro, avocado, salsa, and lime juice in a big bowl. Pour salsa and lime juice over mixture and toss evenly. Separate into two separate ramekin dishes and top with the avocado and cilantro. You may serve with a dollop of vegan sour cream.

Vegetarian Cabbage Rolls

1 head of green cabbage, steamed until leaves are soft
2 cups of cooked quinoa
1 cup of cooked lentils (if using canned, choose organic)
2 cups of finely chopped spinach or Swiss chard
1 small white onion, chopped
1 garlic clove, minced
1 tbsp of coconut oil
1 tsp of dried rosemary
2 tbsp of freshly chopped parsley
Sea salt and pepper to taste
3 cups of Mama's marinara sauce

In a large bowl, combine the quinoa, lentils, spinach, rosemary, parsley, salt and pepper. Toss well.

Using a small frying pan, heat coconut oil on medium heat and sauté garlic and onions until soft. Add this mixture to your bowl and toss again.

Preheat oven to 375 Fahrenheit.

Begin gently removing the leaves from the cabbage. Once all leaves are peeled off, place about ½ cup of mixture inside the leaves, fold both ends in, roll tightly.

Pour a layer of Mama's marinara sauce on the bottom of a large glass pan. Place rolls on top of the sauce, neatly in a row. Pour the remaining Mama's marinara sauce on top, generously covering all the cabbage rolls. For a spicier kick, top with red chili flakes. Bake for 40 to 50 minutes or until cabbage leaves are tender.

Tempeh Asian Stir-fry

Serves 2

Marinade

4 oz. (30 ml) of plain tempeh (use organic tofu as alternative)
2 cloves of garlic, minced
¼ cup of tamari or coconut aminos
1 tbsp of organic rice vinegar

1 tsp of turmeric
3 tsp of fresh, grated ginger
2 tsp of brown rice syrup or honey
2 cups of organic broccoli, chopped
1 cup of grated carrot
1 cup of beansprouts
1 organic red bell pepper, sliced into strips
1 cup of organic baby corn
1 tbsp of virgin coconut oil
1 tbsp of chopped green onion

The night before, cut the tempeh into slices or cubes (whichever size you like), and place in a bowl or baggie.
In a separate bowl, combine the marinade ingredients and mix well.
Pour marinade into the bowl or baggie of tempeh and toss until tempeh is coated. This should be left to marinate for at least 12 hours.
Once marinated, heat coconut oil on medium heat until melted.
Add in tempeh along with the marinade, broccoli, carrots, bell pepper, and baby corn.
Lightly stir to coat all the vegetables in the coconut oil and marinade. (You may need to add a few tablespoons of water if the marinade begins to evaporate too much.)
Allow the vegetables to cook for about 7 to 10 minutes or until slightly crunchy.
Once the vegetables are almost cooked, add in the bean sprouts.
Stir and continue to cook for another minute.
Evenly distribute stir-fry in two separate bowls. Top with the chopped green onion.

Side dishes

Mushroom Risotto

3 tbsp of virgin coconut oil
3 small garlic cloves, minced
1 medium yellow onion, chopped
1½ cups of short grain brown rice
2 cups of mushrooms, sliced
5 cups of vegetable broth
½ cup of nutritional yeast
2 tbsp of gluten-free soy sauce
¼ cup white wine
2 tbsp fresh parsley, chopped
Sea salt and pepper to taste

Preheat the oven to 375 degrees Fahrenheit.

Heat 1 tbsp of coconut oil in a large baking pot (with lid). Add in onions and garlic, sauté until onions are translucent.

Add 4 cups of the vegetable broth and bring to a boil.

Remove from heat, pour in rice, and stir. Cover and bake for about 65 minutes or until rice is tender.

Heat 2 tbsp of coconut oil in a pan. Sautee mushrooms and parsley for about 5 minutes, until mushrooms are soft.

Remove pot from the oven. Add in the mushrooms, white wine, gluten-free soy sauce, nutritional yeast, and salt and pepper. Stir well until all ingredients are combined.

Divide into bowls and top with fresh parsley

Cauliflower Sweet Potato Mash (mashed potato substitute)

3 to 4 cloves of garlic, crushed, then minced

2 large sweet potatoes

1 large head of cauliflower

4 tbsp of virgin coconut oil

Organic vegetable broth (low sodium)

4 tbsp of fresh chives

Sea salt and pepper to taste

In a small frying pan, melt a tsp of coconut oil on medium heat. Sauté garlic until slightly crispy and brown.

Slice sweet potatoes into 2-inch thick wedges and place in a steamer. Next, roughly chop the cauliflower head and place on top of the sweet potato. If you are using a steamer, you will have to let the vegetables cook for 45 minutes to an hour or until soft and tender.

In a food processor or high-speed blender, purée the steamed cauliflower and sweet potato, roasted garlic, salt and pepper, and the remaining coconut oil. If the mixture is too thick, add in enough vegetable broth until you have a smooth consistency. (Unless you like chunks.)

Spoon out into a glass dish and top with chives. Place glass dish in the oven and broil until golden brown.

Maple-glazed Roasted Yams

4 cups of sliced yams

1 tbsp of melted virgin coconut oil

2 tbsp of pure maple syrup

¼ tsp of cayenne pepper

Tbsp of fresh lemon juice

Sea salt and pepper to taste

Preheat oven to 425 degrees Fahrenheit. Line baking sheet or large glass pan with parchment paper.

In a large bowl, mix coconut oil, lemon juice, cayenne pepper, and maple syrup.

Add in your carrots and toss well to coat every carrot evenly.

Place yams on baking sheet and sprinkle with salt and pepper,

Roast the yams for 20 to 30 minutes (depending on how thick your yams are cut), flipping them over half way (at 10 to 15 minutes).

Your yams are cooked when pierced easily with a fork

Salads

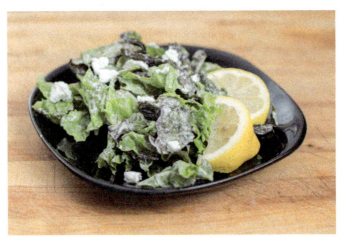

You come first photography

Salad In A Jar

The best way to pack your lunch!

What you will need:

1. A mason jar or any type of large glass jar with a lid

2. Some leafy greens, such as kale, spinach, romaine, green leaf lettuce, etc.

3. A big handful of crunchy veggies! Carrots, onion, cucumber, bell peppers, avocado, etc.

4. Yummy toppings. Nuts, seeds, dried fruit, nutritional yeast.

5. A filling grain or protein! Quinoa, brown rice, beans, sweet potato, free-range chicken, etc.

6. Dressing! Choose a non-dairy, gluten-free, organic dressing or make your own using flax or avocado oil, lemon juice, or some balsamic vinegar. Salsa makes a great dressing too!

How you prepare it:
Start by always pouring a desired amount of dressing at the bottom of the jar.
Next, throw in some of those crunchy veggies! (Not the leafy greens)
After the veggies, comes the grains or protein, or both!
Then, you want to pack in your leafy greens. This should be the main staple in your meal.
To top it all off, add a bit of a kick with some lovely seeds or raisins.
Now for the fun part. When you are ready to eat, simply tip your jar upside down and let the dressing make its way through all your layers until your creative piece of art in a jar becomes your delicious salad. Preparing your salad this way prevents unwanted sogginess and far less Tupperware. Plus, it just looks cool!
Don't feel like getting creative? Try one of my delicious concoctions!

Greek Goddess

1st layer (bottom): Splash of olive oil, red wine vinegar, lemon juice, and a pinch of sea salt and Greek seasoning
2nd layer: Chopped red onion, tomato, and cucumber
3rd layer: Chopped romaine lettuce
4th layer: Black olives, organic goat's milk feta cheese

Garden of Green

1st layer (bottom): Splash of balsamic vinegar, apple cider vinegar, and avocado or flax seed oil
2nd layer: Diced Bartlett pears, cucumber, and zucchini
3rd layer: cooked quinoa (cook quinoa in veggie broth instead of water for more flavour)
4th layer: Spinach
5th layer: Organic goat cheese and walnut crumbs

Kale-fornia Love

1st layer (bottom): Extra virgin olive oil, splash of fresh orange and lemon juice, tsp of raw honey or brown rice syrup
2nd layer: Orange segments, red onion, red bell pepper, peas
3rd layer: Cooked chickpeas
4th layer: Torn kale leaves (discard the stems)

5th layer: Chopped, pitted dates, hulled hemp hearts, and pumpkin seeds (raw)

Mexi Mix

1st layer (bottom): Mama's salsa (see recipe), squirt of lime juice, dash of Cajun spice, splash of hot sauce (optional)
2nd layer: Diced tomato, corn, cucumber, green and yellow bell pepper, avocado
3rd layer: Cooked black beans
4th layer: Arugula or spinach leaves

Everything Salad

5 cups of your favourite organic, leafy, greens. I love using a blend of different greens.
½ ripe avocado
1 carrot, grated
¼ cup of corn kernels
¼ cup of peas
½ red bell pepper, sliced
¼ cup of red onion, minced
6 chopped dates
½ cup baked yam

Dressing
2 tbsp of raw apple cider vinegar
1 tbsp of tamari
Juice from half a lemon
Sea salt and pepper
In a large salad bowl, combine all ingredients, except for dressing and toss well so the avocado and yam become slightly pureed and coat the vegetables. In a small bowl, whisk the dressing ingredients well. Pour over salad and toss again. Serve with a sprig of fresh parsley for garnish.

Raw Caesar Salad

1 head of romaine lettuce, chopped
½ ripe tomato, cut into chunks
1 tbsp of raw seeds (pumpkin, sunflower, hemp, etc.)
¼ cup of raw Caesar dressing (see recipe)
2 tsp of fresh lemon juice

In a large salad bowl, combine romaine lettuce, tomato, and pumpkin seeds, and then toss with raw Caesar dressing and lemon juice. Serve with a slice of fresh lemon.

Baby Kale Cashew Salad with Organic Goat Cheese

4 cups of organic baby kale
½ cup sliced red pepper
¼ cup of crushed raw cashews
1 tbsp of crumbled organic goat cheese
1 tbsp of juice-sweetened cranberries
2 tbsp of balsamic vinegar
2 tbsp of avocado or flaxseed oil

In a large salad bowl, combine all ingredients except for goat cheese. Toss well so dressing coats the salad evenly. Top with goat cheese

Soups and stews

Free-range Chicken and Kale Noodle Soup

3 large, organic chicken breast fillets, cut into thin slices
1 tbsp of coconut oil
2 celery stalks, diced
1 large yellow onion, chopped
2 large carrots, grated
2 garlic cloves, minced
3 cups of kale, finely chopped with stems removed
6 cups of organic, low-sodium chicken broth
8 oz. (226 grams) of gluten-free macaroni or rotini noodles
1 tsp of smoked paprika
Black pepper to taste

In a large pot, melt coconut oil on medium heat. Brown the chicken for about 5 minutes.
Add in the onion and sauté until transparent.
Pour in the chicken broth and bring to a boil.
Reduce heat, and then add in the remaining ingredients.

Thai Coconut Curry

1 tbsp of virgin coconut oil
1 medium yellow onion, diced
1 tsp of organic, ground ginger
3 large garlic cloves minced
1 yellow pepper, sliced thin
½ cup of grated carrots
1 green bell pepper, sliced
½ cup broccoli florets
2 cans of full-fat coconut milk
1 tbsp of red curry powder
¾ cup of organic, low-sodium vegetable broth
Fresh basil to garnish
Sea salt and black pepper to taste
Cooked brown rice or quinoa to serve

In a large pan, melt coconut oil on medium heat. Add onions, garlic, peppers, carrots, and broccoli florets. Saute until somewhat tender. Add in the coconut milk, vegetable broth, curry powder, ginger, sea salt, and pepper and stir. Bring to a boil, then reduce heat and let simmer for about 10 minutes until vegetables are soft. Serve over brown rice or quinoa and top with fresh basil leaves

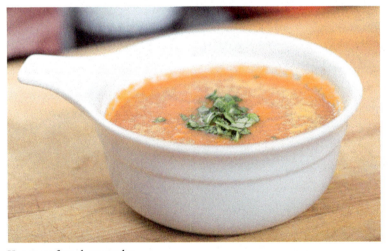

You come first photography

***Roasted Red Pepper Tomato and Basil Soup

1 organic red pepper
3 large, ripe tomatoes

1 small white onion, diced

1 28 oz. (3.5 cups) can of diced tomatoes

1 tbsp of virgin coconut oil

3 heaping tbsp of organic tomato paste

1½ cups of organic low-sodium vegetable broth

½ ripe avocado

4 large basil leaves, stems removed

Sea salt and pepper to taste

Preheat oven to 375 degrees Fahrenheit.

Core the pepper and slice into thick slices. Cut the tomatoes, garlic, and onions in quarters and place in a large bowl along with the peppers. Drizzle with melted coconut oil and toss until evenly coated. Sprinkle with sea salt and pepper and toss again.

Spread vegetable mixture evenly on baking sheet and roast for

35 to 40 minutes or until vegetables are tender.

In a large pot, bring vegetable broth, basil leaves, salt and pepper to a boil.

Add in the canned tomatoes, tomato paste, and the roasted vegetables.

Reduce heat to low and simmer for 15 minutes.

Remove pot from heat and allow to slightly cool for 10 minutes.

Pour soup into a food processor or high-speed blender for 90 seconds. Add in the avocado flesh and purée for 60 seconds or until smooth.

Serve warm.

Apple Squash Bisque

2 cups of butternut squash, seeded, peeled, and diced into cubes

1 organic gala apple, peeled and cored, sliced into wedges

2 tbsp of virgin coconut oil

1 large white onion, diced

5 large garlic cloves, minced

1 cup of organic carrots, chopped

3 cups of organic, low-sodium chicken or vegetable broth

1 cup of unsweetened, plain almond milk

1 tbsp of fresh ginger, peeled and grated

1 tsp of fresh turmeric, peeled and grated

Toasted pine nuts for garnish

Sea salt and pepper to taste

In a large pot, heat olive oil on medium heat and sauté the garlic, onion, turmeric, and ginger.

Add in the broth and almond milk and bring to a boil.

Reduce the heat to low then add in the squash, apple, and carrot.

Simmer for 20 to 25 minutes or until squash is soft.

Add in the sea salt and pepper. Stir well.

Remove pot from heat and allow to cool for 15 minutes.

Pour soup mixture into a food processor or high-speed blender and purée for 90 seconds until smooth.

Top with toasted pine nuts.

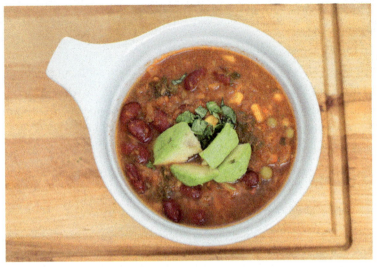

You come first photography

***Mama's Tangy Crockpot Chili

Serves 8

2 tsp of coconut oil

1 medium onion, finely chopped

2 large carrots, chopped

1 green bell pepper, diced

1 yellow pepper, diced

5 large mushrooms, diced

1 cup of organic corn kernels

3 garlic cloves, minced

2 celery stalks, diced

2 cans of organic green chili peppers

3 cans of diced or crushed organic tomatoes (you may also use equivalent of Mama's marinara sauce to opt for a homemade sauce)

¼ cup of chili powder

2 tbsp of dried oregano

1 can of organic black beans, drained and rinsed

1 can of organic red kidney beans, drained and rinsed

Sea salt, pepper, and nutritional yeast to taste

In a small saucepan, heat coconut oil on medium heat.

Add in onions and garlic and sauté until soft.

In a large crockpot or slow cooker, add in all the ingredients including the onion and garlic mixture. Cook on high for about 6 hours or until vegetables are very tender.

Let cool and top with fresh avocado slices and nutritional yeast before serving.

Slow cooker Organic Bison Stew

2 lbs (aprox 3..5 cups) of bison roast
1 medium yellow onion, diced
3 garlic cloves, minced
2 celery sticks, diced
½ cup mushrooms diced
2 large carrots, diced
4¼ cups of organic, low-sodium beef broth
5 baby red potatoes cut in quarters
¼ cup of gluten-free flour
1 6 oz (aprox 3/4 cup) can of organic tomato paste
1 cup of green beans, chopped
1 tbsp of dried parsley
1 tsp of dried rosemary
1 tsp dried oregano
1 tbsp of tamari sauce
Sea salt and pepper to taste

Combine all ingredients into a slow cooker. Cook on high for 7-8 hours.

Desserts

Coconut Maceroons

Ingredients
1 cup of unsweetened coconut, shredded
1 tbsp of almond flour
½ cup coconut milk
½ tsp of pure vanilla extract
1 tbsp of brown rice syrup

Preheat oven to 350 degrees Fahrenheit. Line a baking sheet with parchment paper. Combine all ingredients in a small saucepan over medium heat. Cook, stirring frequently, about 3 minutes or until mixture thickens. Remove from heat and let cool slightly. Once easily handled, place 1 packed tbsp of mixture onto baking sheet. Place in oven on middle rack and cook 20 to 22 minutes until lightly golden. Let cool completely.

Super Easy Raw Chocolate Truffles

1 cup pitted medjool dates (soaked in water overnight)
¼ cup of chia seeds
1 tbsp of raw carob or pure cocoa powder
Additional cocoa powder to dust
Combine all ingredients in a food processor and purée until a smooth batter has formed. Scoop tsp amounts of batter and roll into balls. Coat balls in hemp seeds and place evenly on a parchment paper lined baking tray. Place truffle tray in the freezer for 1 hour to set.

Whipped Pumpkin Mousse

1 block of firm silken organic tofu
1 cup of pure pumpkin puree
¼ cup of pure maple syrup
3 tsp of powdered stevia
1 tsp of pure vanilla extract
1 tsp of pumpkin pie spice (see recipe below)
Coconut whipped cream (see recipe)
Chopped walnuts to garnish
Place all ingredients into a food processor for about 90 seconds until smooth. Divide mousse into fancy glasses and top with a dollop of coconut whipped cream (see recipe) and top with chopped walnuts.

Pumpkin Pie Spice

4 tsp cinnamon
4 tsp of ground ginger
4 tsp of ground nutmeg
3 tsp of allspice
In a small bowl, combine all spices and mix well.

Date Rice Crispy Balls

4 oz. (approx ½ cup) of earth balance or coconut butter
½ cup of brown rice syrup
½ cup of chopped, raw walnuts
1 cup of pitted dates (soaked overnight)
1 cup of unsweetened, shredded coconut
1 tsp of pure vanilla extract
3 cups of brown crispy rice (like Rice Krispies™) cereal

In a small glass bowl, combine the earth balance or coconut butter with the brown rice syrup and vanilla and microwave for 15 seconds or until melted.
Pour syrup mixture into a large bowl.
Add in the walnuts, dates, and coconut, and mix well.
Combine 3 cups of the crispy rice cereal into the large bowl and mix well until thick dough is formed.
Take the remaining cup of crispy rice cereal and place in food processor or high-speed blender. Pulse for a few seconds until the crispy rice cereal is somewhat crushed and spread out on baking sheet. (Do not over-pulse into a powder.)
Place dough mixture in freezer for one hour to slightly harden.
Scoop dough using an ice cream scoop and roll into tbsp size balls.
Roll balls in the remaining crushed crispy rice cereal.

*Chocolate Avocado Pudding

1 medium, ripe avocado
2 tbsp of unsweetened, raw cocoa powder or carob powder
2 tablespoons of pure maple syrup or stevia to taste
5 tbsp of coconut milk or cream
1 tbsp of crushed pistachio nuts or shredded unsweetened coconut

Cut the avocado in half, and scoop its flesh out into a food processor, discarding the pit. Add in the other ingredients, except the pistachios/coconut, and pulse until pudding smooth. Scrape out pudding using a rubber spatula into 2 small ramekins. Top with crushed pistachios or coconut.

Monkey's Ice Cream

2 large bananas, frozen
1 cup of your favourite fruit, frozen
1 to 2 tbsp of unsweetened almond or coconut milk

Place all ingredients in a food processor or high-speed blender and blend until a smooth ice cream consistency is formed. You may need to add more or less milk, depending on thick you like your ice cream. Top your ice cream with cinnamon, slivered almonds, raw carob chips, or more fresh fruit. For a different twist, replace 1 cup of your favourite frozen fruit with 1 tbsp of raw cocoa powder or natural peanut butter!

<u>Cinnamon Brown Rice Pudding</u>

1½ cups of brown basmati rice

1/3 cup of coconut palm sugar or 15 drops of liquid stevia (use more or less depending on level of sweetness preferred)

1 tsp of pure vanilla or caramel extract

Pinch of sea salt

7 cups of organic, unsweetened coconut milk (not cream)

1 pear sliced in wedges

1 tbsp of cinnamon, plus more for garnish

Brown rice syrup or raw honey (optional)

In a large pot, add 4 cups of coconut milk, 1 tbsp of cinnamon, salt, vanilla, and sugar or stevia. Bring to a boil then immediately reduce to low heat and simmer until milk has been absorbed. Add 2 more cups of coconut milk and stir.

Once the last 2 cups of milk have been absorbed, add the last cup of coconut milk, and stir. Spoon into ramekin dishes and top with sliced pear, cinnamon, and a drizzle of brown rice syrup or honey.

Breezy Banana Pecan Bread

½ cup of rolled oats

½ cup of brown rice four

¼ cup of almond or coconut flour

1 tbsp of cornstarch

Pinch of baking soda

½ tsp of baking powder

1 tsp of cinnamon

1/3 cup of chopped pecans

Pinch of sea salt

3 very ripe mashed bananas

¼ cup of homemade vanilla almond or hemp milk (see recipe)

2 tsp of coconut oil

1 tsp of pure vanilla extract

Stevia to taste

Preheat oven to 360 degrees Fahrenheit.

In a large bowl, add the mashed bananas along with the wet ingredients
In another bowl, mix the dry ingredients together. Then
combine the dry and the wet ingredients. Mix well.
Spoon out batter in a non-stick pan.
Bake for 45 minutes or until a fork comes out clean.

Condiments and dressing

Mama's Tomato Sauce

½ large onion, diced
3 garlic cloves, minced
4 large, organic tomatoes
½ tsp garlic powder
¼ tsp onion powder
½ tsp dried oregano or a sprig fresh
4 fresh basil leaves, pressed than minced
Sea salt and pepper

Place about ¼ cup water in a large pot on medium heat and sauté onions and garlic until soft. Add in all the remaining ingredients and simmer for about 15 minutes. For a spicier kick, try adding in some cayenne pepper or red chili flakes. Store in a glass mason jar in the refrigerator

Mama's Salsa

4 large, ripe, organic tomatoes, diced
½ large red onion, chopped
2 cups of chopped cilantro
1 yellow bell pepper, diced
½ cup of organic corn kernels
1 small can of green crushed chili peppers
Sea salt and pepper to taste
Juice of 1 lime

Combine all diced vegetables in a bowl. Toss in the lime juice and the salt and pepper until coated evenly. I also love to add some diced avocado right into the salsa. Just be sure to seal in an air-tight container, as the avocado will turn brown. Store in a glass mason jar in the refrigerator

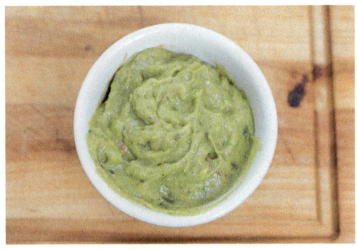

You come first photography

Mama's Guacamole

  3 ripe avocados, flesh and pit removed (save the pit)
  1 red bell pepper, finely chopped
  1 ripe tomato, roughly chopped
  ½ cup cilantro, minced
  Juice of 1 lime
  ½ large red onion, finely chopped
  1 jalapeno pepper, finely chopped (optional)
  Sea salt and pepper to taste

In a large bowl, mash the avocado with a whisk or potato masher. Mash less for a chunkier guacamole or mash more for a creamier, smoother guacamole. Add in the fresh lime juice, sea salt, and pepper and toss. Add in the remaining ingredients and mix well. To store, spoon guacamole into a container, place the avocado stone on top, and seal the container with an airtight lid. The avocado pit prevents the guacamole from browning. Store in the refrigerator

Raw Creamy Ranch Dressing

  1 cup of raw cashews (soaked overnight)
  ¼ cup of raw organic apple cider vinegar
  3 tbsp of fresh lemon juice
  2 garlic cloves
  Pinch of stevia powder

1 tbsp of Mrs. Dash or Herbamare
½ tsp of dried dill
1 large carrot, peeled and chopped
1 tbsp of chopped green onion
½ cup of water or plain almond milk

Place all ingredients in a food processor or high-speed blender and purée until smooth. Store in the refrigerator in a glass jar.

Honey Avocado Mustard Dressing

1 ripe avocado, pitted and flesh removed
1 tbsp of fresh lemon juice
1 tbsp of raw honey
¼ tsp of organic mustard powder
3 tbsp of raw apple cider vinegar
Sea salt and pepper to taste

Place all ingredients in a food processor or high-powered blender and purée until smooth. Store in the refrigerator in a glass jar.

Raw Cole slaw dressing

1/3 cup of raw cashews (soaked overnight)
3 table spoons of raw pumpkin seeds
1 tbsp of raw apple cider vinegar
1 tsp of stone ground mustard
1 clove of crushed garlic
Sea salt and pepper to taste
½ tsp of paprika
3 tbsp of fresh lemon juice
2 tbsp of nutritional yeast
½ cup of water (add more for a thinner dressing)

Place all ingredients in a food processor or high-speed blender and purée until smooth. Store in the refrigerator in a glass jar.

Gluten-free BBQ Sauce

1 5 oz. (just over 1/2 cup) can of organic tomato paste
2 tbsp of organic garlic powder
2 tbsp of organic mustard powder
2/3 cup of raw apple cider vinegar
3 tbsp of maple syrup

1½ tbsp of paprika
Sea salt and pepper to taste
Small pinch of stevia powder
Place all ingredients in a processor or high-speed blender and purée until smooth. Store in the refrigerator in a glass jar.

RAW Alfredo Sauce

½ cup of raw cashews (soaked overnight)
2 tsp of organic garlic powder
1 tbsp
1 tsp of tamari
2 tbsp of nutritional yeast
½ cup of water or dairy-free milk (add more to thin)
Sea salt and pepper to taste
Place ingredients in a high-speed blender for 90 seconds until smooth. Store in a glass mason jar in the fridge. (Also freezes well.)

Raw Caesar Salad Dressing

1/3 cup of raw cashews or macadamia nuts (soaked overnight)
2 tbsp of fresh lemon juice
1 tsp of tamari sauce
1 to 2 tsp of organic garlic powder
Sea salt and pepper to taste
¼ cup of unsweetened almond milk (add more to thin)
1 to 2 tbsp of nutritional yeast
In a high-speed blender, purée the ingredients for 90 seconds until smooth. Store in a glass jar in the fridge (Also freezes well.)

Mushroom Gravy

2½ cups of organic, low-sodium vegetable broth
2¼ tbsp of cornstarch
½ cup minced white onion
9 oz. (just over 1 cup) of mushroom of choice, chopped
1 tsp of oregano
1 tsp of rosemary

1 tsp of Dijon mustard

2 tbsp nutritional yeast

3 tbsp of white wine

1 tbsp of tamari or coconut aminos

Salt and pepper to taste

Tsp of coconut oil

In a large pan, heat coconut oil on medium heat. Add in onions, garlic, and mushrooms and sauté until onions are translucent.

Pour in the vegetable broth along with the oregano and rosemary. Let simmer for about 2 minutes on low heat.

In a separate bowel, whisk the wine, tamari, yeast, Dijon mustard, and cornstarch until it becomes a thick and smooth paste.

Add the paste to the broth mixture and whisk continuously until gravy is thick. (It will only take a couple of minutes. If the gravy becomes too thick, add more vegetable broth.)

Finally, add in the salt and pepper, whisk one more time.

Serve over mashed potatoes, vegetables, meat, or vegetarian dishes.

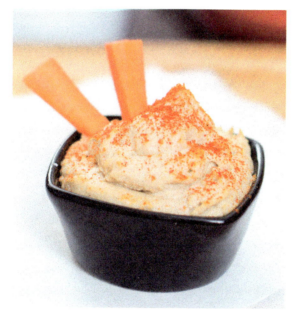

You come first photography

*Traditional Hummus

2 cups of cooked or canned chickpeas, rinsed

2 heaping tbsp of organic tahini

4 to 5 tbsp of extra virgin olive or flax seed oil

Juice of 1 large lemon

1 garlic clove or 2 tsp of garlic powder

Sea salt and pepper to taste

5 tbsp of water (add more for a creamier humus)

Place all ingredients in a food processor or high-speed blender and purée until smooth. Store in an airtight container in the refrigerator

Snacks

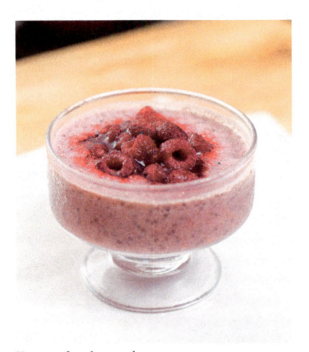

You come first photography

***Vanilla Raspberry Chia Pudding**

1 cup of homemade vanilla almond or hemp milk

2 tbsp of pure maple syrup

2 dates (soaked overnight)

1 tsp of pure vanilla extract

¼ cup of organic chia seeds

2 cups of fresh raspberries

Raspberries and mint leaves for garnish

In a large bowl, combine almond or hemp milk and chia seeds and stir. Let stand for about an hour or until the chia seeds have absorbed all the milk and create a gel.

In a food processor or high-speed blender, purée the remaining ingredients (not the chia gel) until smooth.
Combine the raspberry chocolate purée with the chia gel and mix well.
Spoon the chia pudding in decorative bowls and top with fresh raspberries and mint leaves.

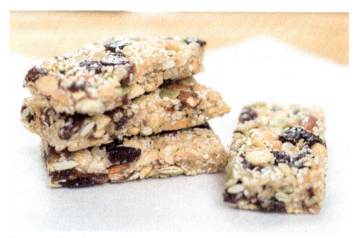

You come first photography

***Mama's Granola Bars**

2 cups of rolled, gluten-free oats
½ cup pumpkin seeds
½ cup slivered almonds
½ cup chia seeds
½ cup hemp or sesame seeds
Heaping ½ cup of raisins or chopped dates
Pinch of sea salt
1 tsp of cinnamon
1 tsp of pure vanilla extract
1½ cups of mashed, ripe bananas

Preheat oven to 375 degrees Fahrenheit. Coat a large glass baking pan with a small amount of coconut oil, then line your pan with a layer of parchment paper to prevent the bars from sticking.
Place all dry ingredients except for the raisins/dates in a food processor or blender, and pulse until slightly chopped. (Don't pulse for too long as the mixture will become flour.)
In a large bowl, combine your oat mix with the mashed bananas, raisins, and vanilla.
Mix well until all wet and dry ingredients become a dough-like texture.
Spoon mixture into your pan and smooth out with a spatula.
Bake for 20 to 25 minutes, until the top layer is slightly golden and crisp.

Let cool for 10 minutes before removing the bars from the pan. Place on a breadboard for cooling, and refrigerate for 1 to 2 hours until bars are firm and cool. Slice the bars and enjoy!

Oatmeal Raisin Cookies

3 ripe bananas, mashed
2 cups of rolled oats
1/3 cup of organic applesauce
¼ cup of coconut, rice, or almond milk (unsweetened)
1 tsp of nutmeg
1 tsp of cinnamon
1 tsp of pure vanilla extract
1 tbsp of ground flax seeds
½ cup soaked raisins (place raisins in 1 cup of hot water, soak for 30 minutes, then drain)
Preheat oven to 350 degrees Fahrenheit.
In a large bowl, mash peeled bananas with a fork or potato masher until smooth.
Add in the applesauce, vanilla, cinnamon, nutmeg, flax, and vanilla, and stir.
Fold in the oats and raisins.
Using an ice cream scoop or tablespoon, spoon dough balls onto an ungreased cookie sheet.
Bake cookies 15 to 20 minutes until golden brown. Cool before serving

Raw Trail Mix

1 cup of raw walnuts (soaked overnight), chopped
1 cup of raw, slivered almonds
½ cup of dried raisins
½ cup of dry apple rings, chopped
½ cup dates, pitted and chopped
½ cup chia seeds
½ cup hemp seeds
1 tsp of cinnamon
2 tbsp of pure maple syrup or brown rice syrup
In a large bowl, combine all the ingredients and mix well
until syrup has coated the entire mixture.
Spread the mixture out evenly on a mesh dehydrator tray and dehydrate for 5 to 6 hours or until dry and crunchy. If no dehydrator is available, spread mixture out on a parchment paper lined baking sheet, and bake for 2 hours at 100 degrees Fahrenheit, or until dry and crunchy. Serve on top of dairy-free yogurt or eat as is for a light, on-the-go snack!

Super Food Energy Balls

These little energy balls are calorie-dense and perfect for before or after a workout. Chock-full of super foods and nutrients, they will become your go-to snack for an afternoon pick-me-up!

12 to 15 dates (soaked overnight)

1/3 cup of walnut crumbs

1/3 cup of raisins or goji berries

2 tbsp of hemp hearts

1 tsp of pure vanilla extract

1 tbsp of maca powder (found at health stores; optional)

2 tbsp of raw cocoa nibs

½ tbsp of brown rice syrup

Shredded, unsweetened coconut and pure cocoa powder for garnish

Combine all ingredients in a food processor and purée until a smooth batter forms.

Dip your hands in lukewarm water and scoop out tablespoons of dough. Roll into small balls.

Sprinkle coconut and cocoa powder on parchment paper and

coat balls until they are no longer sticky to the touch.

Place balls in freezer for an hour to harden.

Store in the refrigerator in an airtight container or bag

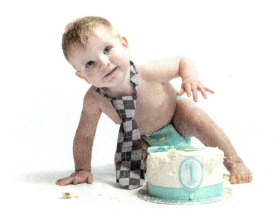

JM Photography

Baby food Recipes

I absolutely love making baby food from scratch. You know exactly what ingredients are going into it and you can be reassured that there are no preservatives. Preparing and storing your own baby food is quite simple, not to mention cheaper and healthier than buying store-bought baby food. I've provided my top recipes that my clients' babies just adore! All you will need are the ingredients, a food processor or high-speed blender, a rubber spatula, and an ice tray or baby food storage containers.

Babies 6-8 months old

To prepare these recipes, place all ingredients in a food processor or high-speed blender and purée until smooth. Additional instructions may be added.

Apple of my eye

　　4 large organic gala apples or other sweet apple of choice, peeled and cored and sliced (soaked for 1 hour in hot water prior to blending)
　　Squeeze of organic lemon juice
　　1 to 2 tbsp of organic apple juice if needed to thin

Banana Blueberry Pudding

　　1 very ripe, organic banana
　　1 cup of organic blueberries
　　1 to 2 tbsp of water if needed to thin

Banana Cream Pie

　　1 very ripe, organic banana
　　Squeeze of organic lemon juice
　　½ ripe organic avocado
　　1 to 2 tbsp of water if needed to thin

Peaches and Cream

　　2 cups of organic, ripe peaches, peeled and diced

4 tbsp of breast milk or ready to drink formula
½ ripe, organic banana

Thanksgiving Dinner

1 cup of steamed organic green beans
½ cup organic pumpkin purée (canned is fine)
1 tbsp of chopped, free-range chicken, cooked
2 to 4 tbsp of water or organic chicken stock

A Pea In My Pod

½ cup of steamed organic peas
1 organic pear, peeled, cored, and sliced
1/2 cup of organic, slightly steamed spinach

Strawberry Sunday

1 cup of organic strawberries, stems removed
3 prunes (soaked in hot water for 2 hours)
½ ripe organic banana
1 to 2 tbsp of water if needed to thin

Orange Is The New Pink

½ cup organic baby carrots, steamed
½ cup organic butternut squash, steamed
¼ cup of organic yam, steamed
2 to 4 tbsp of fresh-squeezed orange juice

Green Means Go!

½ organic zucchini, peeled and steamed
½ cup of organic spinach, slightly steamed
½ organic, ripe avocado
1 tbsp of free-range chicken, cooked (optional)
2-3 tbsp of organic beef stock or water

Babies 8-11 months old

At this stage, start processing foods until they are a little bit chunky, but still small enough for baby to easily eat. Introducing new textures is another excellent way to expand baby's palette.
Store baby food in small glass mason jars.

To freeze, pour into plastic ice cube trays and place in the freezer. Remove cubes into a small glass bowl and allow thawing or warming slightly on stove.

Baked Apple Pie

    2 organic gala apples, peeled, cored and sliced (soak in hot water for 1 hour prior to blending)
    Sprinkle of cinnamon
    2 tsp of pure maple syrup
    ½ organic pear, peeled, cored, and sliced

Pumpkin Pie

    1 cup of organic pumpkin purée (canned is fine)
    Pinch of cinnamon
    Pinch of nutmeg
    1 organic, ripe banana
    2 to 4 tbsp of breast milk or ready-to-drink formula or water

Pina Colada

    1 cup of organic pineapple, peeled, cored, and sliced
    1 organic, ripe banana
    1 to 2 tbsp of homemade or unsweetened coconut milk

Magical Melon

    ½ cup of seedless watermelon, flesh removed
    ½ cup organic honey dew, flesh and seeds removed
    ½ cup organic cantaloupe, flesh and seeds removed

Beef Stew

½ cup of organic beef, cooked
½ cup organic carrots, steamed
½ cup organic red potatoes steamed
½ cup of green beans, steamed
2 to 4 tbsp of organic beef stock

Veggie Lentil Soup

½ cup of cooked brown lentils
½ organic raw tomato
¼ cup of organic corn kernels, steamed
½ cup red potatoes, peeled and steamed
1-2 tsp of raw virgin coconut oil
Tbsp of yellow onion, chopped and steamed
2 to 4 tbsp of organic vegetable stock

Quinoa Fruit Porridge

½ cup organic quinoa, cooked
½ cup each of organic blueberries and strawberries
½ cup organic peaches, peeled and sliced
2 tsp of pure maple syrup or 2 dates (soaked in hot water for 1 hour)

Creamy Green Smoothie

1/3 banana
¼ apple, peeled and cored
1 handful of organic kale, stems removed
¼ organic avocado
½ cup coconut water

Cream of Broccoli Soup

½ cup peas, steamed
1 cup of chopped broccoli florets, steamed
1/3 cup of full-fat coconut cream or ½ avocado and 1/3 cup vegetable stock

Pinch of sea salt and garlic powder

Coconut Yogurt Parfait

½ cup of plain coconut yogurt
½ cup of mixed fruit, peeled
¼ avocado
1 to 2 tbsp of breast milk, formula, or dairy-free milk

Toddler Recipes (12 months and up)

You didn't think I would leave out a special recipe section for the toddlers did you? Of course not! Here are some delicious, whole-food meals and snacks to satisfy even the fussiest eater.

Simple Cinnamon Apple Porridge

¼ cup of cooked gluten-free, rolled oats or brown rice
½ cup chopped apple, peeled and cored
Pinch of cinnamon
2 tsp of pure maple syrup
2 to 3 tbsp of homemade vanilla almond or non-dairy milk

Place all ingredients in a food processor or high-speed blender for 90 seconds until smooth.

Apple Wheels

1 apple, seeded and cored
1 to 2 tbsp of almond, peanut, or pumpkin seed butter
1 tbsp of raw cocoa nibs or organic dark chocolate (dairy-free)
1 tbsp of shredded, unsweetened coconut
Sliced apples to create ½ inch rings
Spread rings with the butter of your choice.
Top with shredded coconut and chocolate.

Ants On A Log

2 organic celery sticks, cut in halves
1 tbsp of homemade almond, peanut, or pumpkin seed butter (see recipe)
2 tbsp of organic raisins
Sprinkle of cinnamon
Divide nut or seed butter in half and spread evenly upon celery sticks.
Sprinkle with raisins and cinnamon.

Apple-berry Fruit Rolls

2 apples, peeled and chopped
1 cup of your favourite berries (strawberry, raspberry, blackberry, blueberry, etc.)
Preheat oven to 175 degrees Fahrenheit. Line a cookie sheet with parchment paper.
In a food processor or high-speed blender, purée the
fruits until they have a smooth consistency.
Pour fruit purée onto cookie sheet and evenly spread out the mixture.
Place in the oven for approximately 4 hours until the fruit rolls are dry and not sticky to touch.
Remove from the oven and allow to cool completely. Remove parch-
ment paper from cookie sheet and place on breadboard.
Using a cookie cutter, slice the fruit rolls into long strips.
Use a fresh piece of parchment paper to roll the fruit rolls
to prevent them from sticking together.

Apple Wedges with Dateamel Dip

1 apple, sliced into wedges
½ cup pitted dates
½ tsp of pure vanilla extract
2 to 4 tbsp of water
Soak dates in 2-4 tbsp of hot water overnight until dates are soft and plump.
Pour dates and soaking water into a food processor or high-
speed blender and purée until smooth.
Pour date puree into a small bowl and dip in the apple wedges.

Grilled Greens and Cheese

2 slices of sprouted grain or whole grain gluten-free bread
1 slice of vegan cheese (I love the Daiya brand)

1 to 2 tsp of coconut oil

2 handfuls of spinach or your preferred leafy greens

In a small pan, melt coconut oil on medium heat. Add in the spinach and sauté until tender. Remove the spinach and set aside.

Place the slice of cheese on one of the bread slices and top with the sautéed spinach. Place the other slice of bread on top of the cheese and spinach, creating a sandwich. Place the sandwich in the pan and grill both sides until golden brown and the cheese is melted.

Gluten-free Penne with Lean Green Alfredo Sauce

1 batch of raw Alfredo sauce (see recipe)

4 cups of raw spinach

1 cup of steamed broccoli

Cooked, gluten-free pasta of choice

Black pepper

Dairy/soy-free cheese (such as Daiya)

Combine the spinach and broccoli with one batch of raw Alfredo sauce (see recipe) in a food processor or high-speed blender and purée for about 90 seconds or until smooth. Pour over a bowl of gluten-free pasta and top with freshly ground pepper and shredded, dairy/soy-free cheese.

***Sweet Potato Mac N Cheeze**

1 sweet potato, peeled and cut into 1-inch cubes

½ small onion, finely chopped

½ cup of coconut oil

1 cup of shredded carrots

1 tsp of turmeric

1 tsp of Dijon mustard

½ cup nutritional yeast

3 tbsp of plain almond or hemp milk

2 cups of organic low sodium vegetable broth

Sea salt and pepper to taste

230 g (8 oz) of gluten-free macaroni pasta

Paprika

In a large pot, bring vegetable broth and almond or hemp milk to a boil. Add in the sweet potato, onion, and carrot, and reduce heat to low. Let simmer for about 15 to 20 minutes or until sweet potato is tender.

Pour into a food processor or high-speed blender and purée until smooth. Add in the coconut oil and process again. Add the remaining ingredients except the pasta and process until the sauce is smooth and creamy.

Cook pasta as directed on the box. Strain and pour pasta back into the pot. Combine the sauce with the pasta and mix well. Sprinkle with paprika and additional nutritional yeast if desired.

Raw Chocolate Brownies

2 cups of dates (soaked overnight)
1 cup of raw walnuts (soaked overnight)
1 tbsp of virgin coconut oil
2 tbsp of brown rice syrup or raw honey
3 tbsp of pure cocoa powder
1 tbsp of hemp hearts

Place all ingredients except the hemp hearts in a food processor (this would be a bit more difficult to make in a blender as the dough is really thick) and purée until a smooth batter forms. Line a glass dish with parchment paper to prevent sticking. Pour in brownie mixture and press to create an even surface. Sprinkle with hemp hearts. Place brownies in the freezer for about 90 minutes to set. Once firm, cut into squares using a pizza cutter, and store in the fridge.

Vanilla Bean Cupcakes With Coconut Cream Icing

1 batch of coconut whipped cream (see recipe)
2¼ cups of gluten-free flour (brown rice works well)
1½ cups of coconut palm sugar
½ tsp of baking soda
1 tsp of baking powder
½ cup of melted coconut oil
1½ cups of homemade vanilla almond or hemp milk
2 tsp of pure vanilla extract
1 tbsp of fresh orange juice

Preheat oven to 360 degrees Fahrenheit.

Line muffin tins with parchment paper liners. (I find parchment paper makes the cupcakes much easier to remove from the liner then paper ones.)

In a large bowl, mix together all dry ingredients.

In a smaller bowl, whisk together all the wet ingredients excluding the coconut whipped cream.

Combine wet and dry ingredients and mix well to avoid any clumps.

Pour batter into the lined muffin tins, leaving a 1½ inch space from the top. (The batter will rise slightly, and filling it 2/3 full will prevent spillage and a huge mess!) Bake the cupcakes on the middle rack for 20 to 25 minutes or until a toothpick comes out clean from poking the centre of a cupcake.

Allow cupcakes to cool completely before frosting, as frosting will melt very easily.

To frost, spoon the coconut whipped cream into an icing bag or zip lock. Push the whipped cream to one corner of the back and cut the corner off. Squeeze the whipped cream onto the cupcake in a circular motion to create the "swirl". Top with shredded coconut.

Coconut Whipped Cream

1 can of full-fat coconut milk (do not use light)
1 tsp of pure vanilla extract
2 tsp of powdered stevia
Pinch of cinnamon (optional)

Place can of coconut milk in the refrigerator for 4 hours.

Remove can from refrigerator and flip upside down on counter. This allows for the coconut water to separate from the thick cream.

Using a can opener, remove the lid and drain coconut water into cup. You can either discard the water or save it to add to smoothies and other desserts.

Using a rubber spatula, scoop the thick coconut cream out from the bottom of the can and into a large mixing bowl.

Using a hand-held whisk or electric mixer, whip the coconut cream until fluffy. This usually takes about 1 to 2 minutes.

Store in an airtight container in the refrigerator.

Chapter 17
FITNESS 101: Prenatal and Postnatal Workouts

Keeping active during and after pregnancy is very beneficial to us as mamas and for our little ones! Although most woman do not receive clearance to workout until at least 6 weeks postpartum, planning future workouts is a great way to stay motivated and on track.

I've had the privilege of bringing onboard my personal friend and certified personal trainer, Addrianne Oyewole, who has created a variety of non-generic, very effective exercises that can be done at home or in the gym.

About the trainer

Addrianne Oyewole is all about fitness and health. He is a certified personal trainer and a body-building and fitness professional. He is also the creator of Ufit, a fitness and wellness format, designed to meet the needs of anyone trying to reach their fitness and health goals. Through this format, he has designed different exercises to help expectant and post-partum moms reach their fitness goals without putting any strain on their bodies.

Addrianne has been in the fitness industry for over 12 years and his passion for helping others achieve ultimate health is evident through his exercises. These exercises have been approved to be suitable for postnatal mothers who have given birth naturally or via C-section. As with every new fitness routine, be sure to check with your doctor before starting.

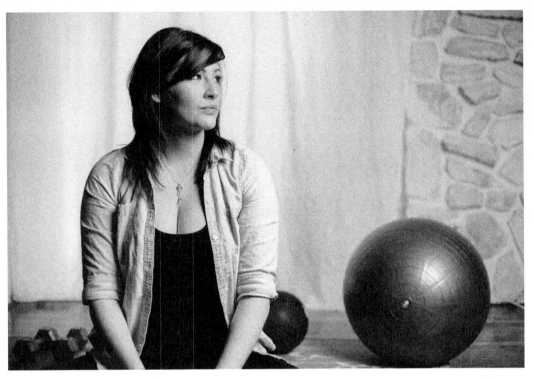

You come first photography

Prenatal exercises

(Can be performed throughout a healthy pregnancy)

Mommies to be! These exercises are targeted for expectant mothers to help increase energy, improve sleep patterns, increase blood flow, reduce stress and joint pain, increase flexibility, and prepare for childbirth.

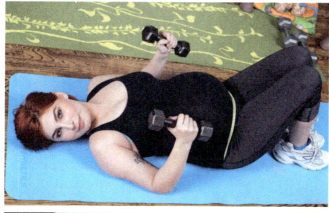

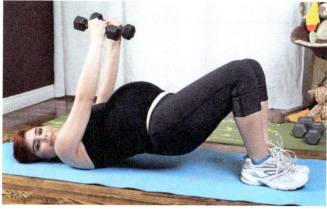

You come first photography

Exercise 1: Modified Glute Bridge

Targets: glutes, hips, lower back, legs, arms, chest

You will need: 2 Dumbbells, yoga mat

10 repetitions/3 sets

Begin by lying flat on your back, knees bent, and heels tucked close to your butt. This is your starting position. While holding a dumbbell in each hand, elbows on the mat, raise your butt up to the celling as far as you can go, while extending your arms straight up. Hold for 3 seconds, and then slowly lower yourself back down onto the mat, bringing your arms back into starting position. Repeat.

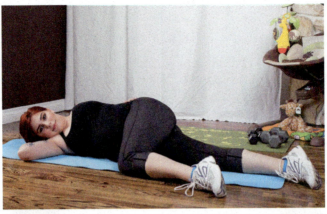

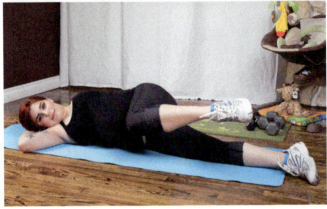

You come first photography

Exercise 2: Lying Hip Flexor
Targets: hips, glutes, legs
You will need: Yoga mat
10 repetitions (each side)/3 sets
Begin by lying on your right side. Place your right arm under your head and your left arm extended behind you. Bring your left leg in front of your right, keeping it slightly bent. This is your starting position. Slowly raise your left leg above the ground, hold for 3 seconds, then bring left leg back down into starting position. Repeat.

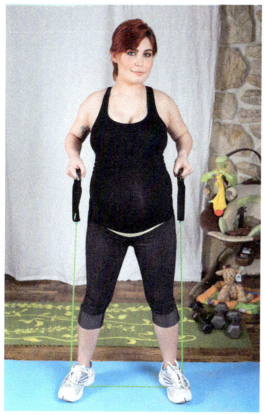 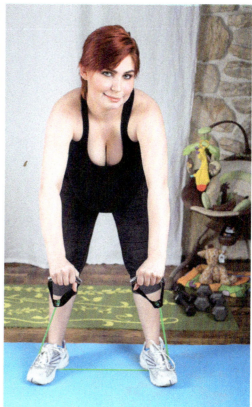

You come first photography

Exercise 3: Modified Standing Row

Targets: back, legs, arms

You will need: A resistance band, yoga mat

10 repetitions/3 sets

Begin by standing with your legs shoulder-width apart with the middle of a resistance band underneath both feet; resistant band handles in each hand. This is your starting position. Pull handles back towards your waist while straightening lower back. Pull shoulders back and push chest forward while arching back. Hold for 2 seconds, then slowly bend slightly forward at the waist, as you extend your arms forward towards the ground. Hold for 2 seconds. Slowly bring yourself back up to starting position. Repeat.

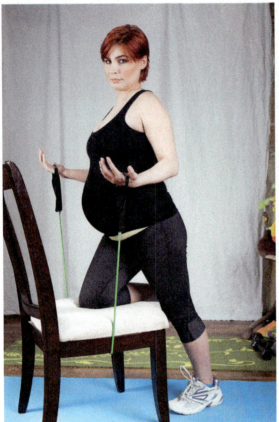 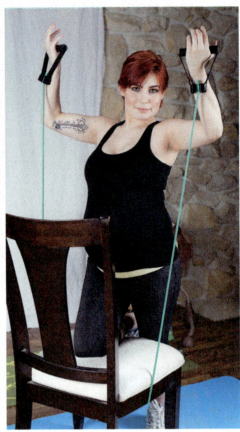

You come first photography

Exercise 4: Open-handed Shoulder Press

Target: arms, shoulders

You will need: a resistant band, a chair

10 repetitions/3 sets

Begin by placing the resistance band underneath the chair. Grab both handles with each hand, placing one knee on a chair facing you and the other foot planted firmly on the floor. This is your starting position. Keeping your abdomen tight, bring both arms up, with your elbows staying at a 90-degree angle. Hold for 2 seconds, then slowly lower arms to starting position.

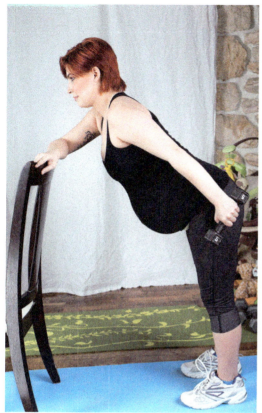 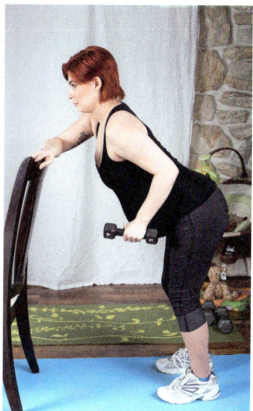

You come first photography

Exercise 5: Chair Modified Triceps Kickback

Target: arms

You will need: 1 dumbbell, a chair

10 repetitions (each side)/3 sets

Begin by turning a chair around so the seat is facing away from you. Place one hand gently on the back of the chair, while the other hand holds a dumbbell. This is your starting position. Keeping your knees slightly bent, extend the arm holding the dumbbell behind you until it is fully straightened (be sure to keep your elbow tucked into your side). Hold for 2 seconds, then slowly bend your arm back to starting position. Repeat.

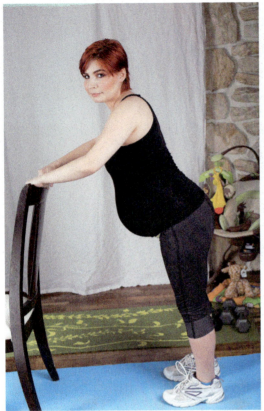 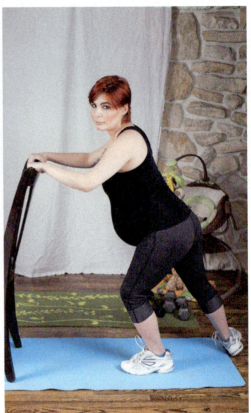

You come first photography

Exercise 6: Modified Chair Hip Flexor

Target: hip flexors, legs, glutes

You will need: a chair

10 repetitions (each side)/3 sets

Begin by turning a chair around so the seat is facing away from you. Place both hands on the back of the chair for support. This is your starting position. Slightly bend your left leg as you fully extend your right leg out to the side, really focusing on squeezing your glutes. Hold for 1 second, then retract your right leg, while straightening your left leg back to the starting position. Repeat.

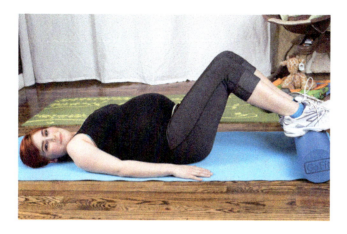

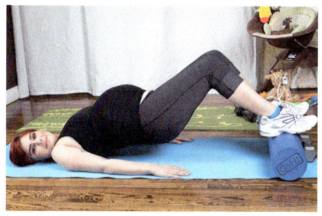

You come first photography

Exercise 7: Modified Glute Bridge with Roller
Targets: glutes, legs, lower back
You will need: Foam roller, yoga mat
10 repetitions/3 sets
Begin by laying flat on your back, knees bent and both feet resting on a foam roller. This is your starting position. Slowly raise your hips off the ground, pressing your feet against the foam roller, focusing on squeezing your glutes. Hold for 2 seconds, and slowly lower back down to starting position. Repeat

Post-natal exercises

(Recommended to begin 6 weeks after birth)

New mommies! These exercises are targeted for post-partum mothers to help promote healthy weight loss, restore muscle tone, increase energy, strengthen abdominal muscles, increase flexibility, and reduce the risk of post-partum depression.

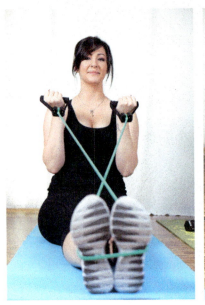 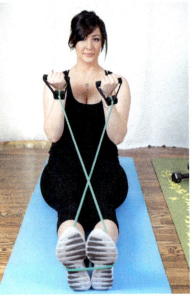

Targets: legs,You come first photography

Exercise 1: Modified Half-bicep Curls
Targets: arms
You will need: 1 exercise band with handles, yoga mat
10 Repetitions/3 Sets
Begin by sitting up straight with your two feet together, legs straight, and abdomen tight. Place middle of the band around your feet, and grab the handles, palms facing up. This is your starting position. Curl your arms up to your chest. Hold for 2 seconds. Slowly bring your arms back down halfway and repeat

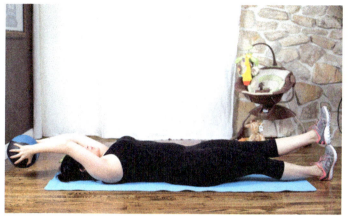
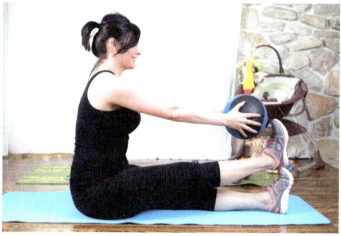

You come first photography

Exercise 3: Abdomen Roll-up with Medicine Ball
Targets: abdominals, lower back, arms
You will need: 5 lb. medicine ball, yoga mat
10 repetitions/3 Sets
Begin by laying flat on your back, holding the medicine ball with your arms extended behind you on the mat, above your head. Rest one heel on top of the other toe. This is your starting position.
Keeping your arms extended, Breath in as you bring your torso up into a sitting position until the medicine ball touches your toes.
(Keep your abdomen tight while performing this exercise.)
As you exhale, slowly bring your torso back on the mat to the starting position. Repeat.

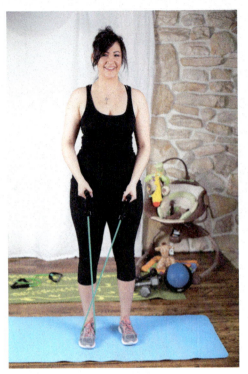 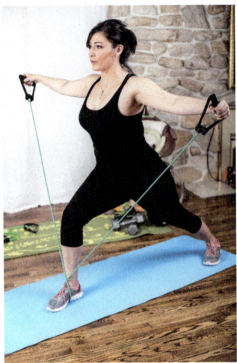

You come first photography

Exercise 4: Lunge with Side Lateral Raise

Targets: legs, glutes, back, abdomen, arms, and shoulders

You will need: 1 resistance band, yoga mat

10 Repetitions (each leg)/3 Sets

Begin by placing the middle of the band underneath one foot. This is your starting position. Stepping back with the opposite leg keeping straight, slowly bend the front leg and lower into lunge position. At the same time, raise arms to sides until elbows are shoulder height. Hold for 2 seconds then slowly release arms down by side, while slowly straightening the front leg and stepping the back leg into starting position. Repeat.

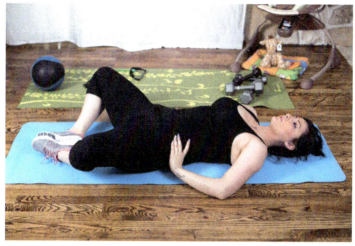

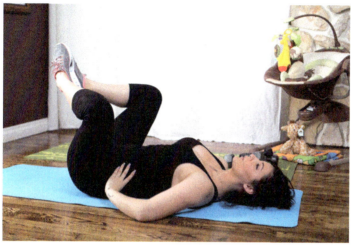

You come first photography

Exercise 5: Reverse Butterfly Crunch

Targets: abdomen

You will need: Yoga mat

10 repetitions/3 Sets

Begin by lying flat on your back, hands on your hips, feet together with your knees bent (try to bring your heels as close to your butt as possible). This is your starting position. Lift your feet off the ground, keeping your bent knee position until you have reached a 90-degree angle. Hold for 3 seconds, then slowly release, holding the same position, back down to the floor. Repeat.

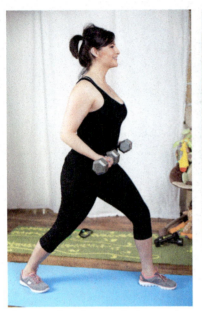 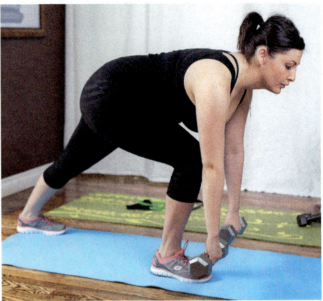

You come first photography

Exercise 6: Altered Deadlift Lunge

Targets: back, abdomen, legs, glutes, arms

You will need: 2 dumbbells, yoga mat

10 Repetitions/3 Sets

Begin by stepping one foot forward and slightly bend at the knee. Elbows bent slightly, holding weights at hip level, palms facing up. This is your starting position.

Slowly begin to drop torso forward, bending at the waist, until your back is flat. At the same time, straighten the arms and reach towards the floor, rotating the wrists so palms face down. Hold for 2 seconds, then slowly rotate wrists back, bending the arms, squeezing shoulder blades together, and bringing the torso back upright and back to starting position. Repeat.

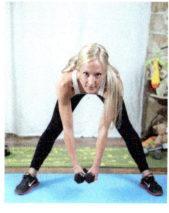 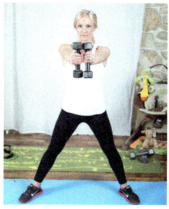
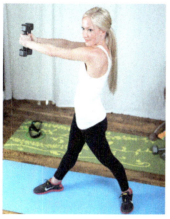 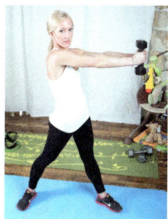

You come first photography

Exercise 7: Wide-stance Dumbbell Swings and Twists
Targets: legs, lower back, arms
You will need: 2 dumbbells, yoga mat
10 repetitions/3 Sets
Begin by standing, legs past shoulder-width apart, torso bent 90 degrees with back straight, arms extended down towards the mat, keeping dumbbells pressed together. This is your starting position.
While keeping dumbbells together, slowly bend torso upright to standing position, keeping arms extended out in front of you and your back straight.
Just using your upper body, twist your torso to the right, keeping arms extended and abdomen tight, and hold for 1 second. Slowly rotate the torso to the left, hold for 1 second, and then bring the torso and arms back to the centre. Hold for 1 second. Slowly bring the torso and arms back into starting position. Repeat.

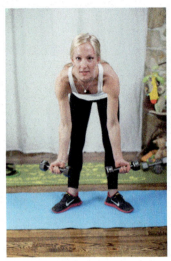 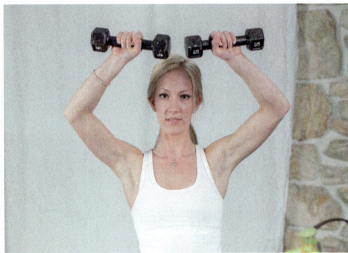

You come first photography

Exercise 8: Revolving Lateral Raise
Targets: back, arms, shoulders
You will need: 2 dumbbells, yoga mat
Begin by standing straight, holding a dumbbell in each hand, elbows bent slightly above your head, palms facing out. This is your starting position. Slowly bring torso downward towards the mat, bending at the hips until a 90-degree angle is reached. Back should be kept flat. At the same time, keeping elbows bent, bring arms down by your side, keeping palms facing outwards. Hold for 2 seconds, and then slowly bring torso to upright position, keeping back straight. At the same time, bring arms back up to the starting position. Repeat.

A Pea in my Pod

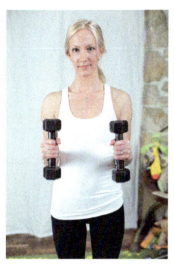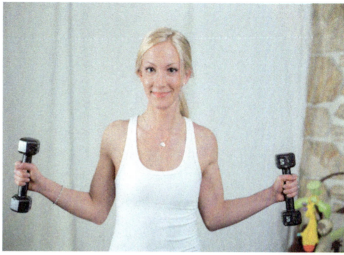

You come first photography

Exercise 9: Dumbbell Rotator Cuff Extension
Targets: rotator cuffs, arms
You will need: 2 dumbbells, yoga mat
10 repetitions/3 Sets
Begin by standing upright, feet shoulder-width apart,
elbows bent. This is your starting position.
Holding a dumbbell in each hand with palms facing together, slowly open your arms out to the sides, keeping your elbows pressed against your sides. Hold for 2 seconds as you extend your chest slightly while squeezing your shoulder blades together. Slowly bring your arms back in to starting position. Repeat.

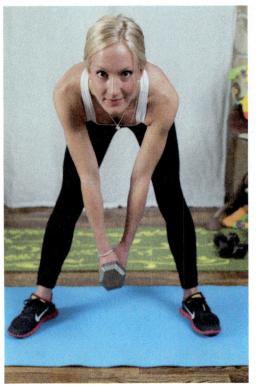
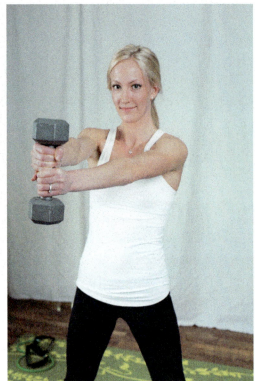

You come first photography

Exercise 10: Dumbbell Back Extension

Targets: lower back, arms, legs

You will need: 1 dumbbell, yoga mat

10 repetitions/3 Sets

Begin standing upright, feet shoulder-width apart, arms extending straight in front of you while holding 1 dumbbell with both hands. This is your starting position. Keep your arms extended, bend your torso downward to the floor until you've reached a 90-degree angle. Hold for 2 seconds, then slowly bring yourself back up into starting position, making sure to keep your back and arms straight. Repeat.

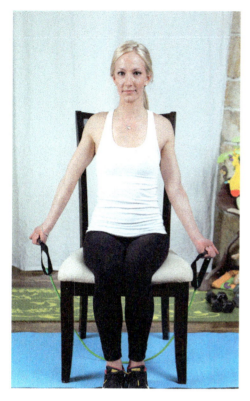 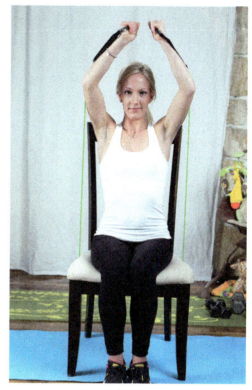

You come first photography

Exercise 11: Seated Shoulder Press

Targets: shoulders, abdomen, arms

You will need: A chair, resistance band

10 repetitions/3 Sets

Begin my placing a resistance band underneath a chair, so the middle of the band meets the middle of the chair seat. Sit on the chair, legs together, holding both handles of the band. This is your starting position. Keep your abdomen tight as you bring both arms up above your head, palms facing inward. Hold for 2 seconds, then slowly bring arms back down into starting position. Repeat.

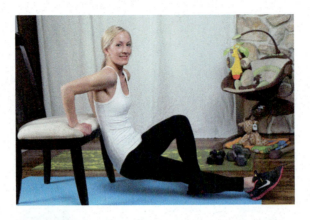

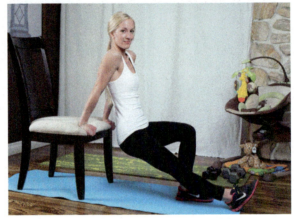

You come first photography

Exercise 12: Chair-assisted Triceps Dip

Targets: arms, back, abdomen

You will need: a chair

10 repetitions/3 Sets

Begin by placing both arms slightly behind you as you hold the edge of your chair, keeping your arms extended. Keep your back as close to the seat of the chair as possible. Extend one leg out in front of you and bend the back leg at a 90-degree angle. This is your starting position.

Slowly begin to bend your elbows to a 90-degree angle and dip your body downward so your butt is almost touching the floor. Hold for 2 seconds, and slowly begin to extend the arms and push yourself back up into starting position. Repeat. (If you find it too difficult to get yourself back up, you may use your bent leg for some assistance.)

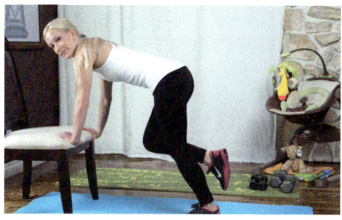

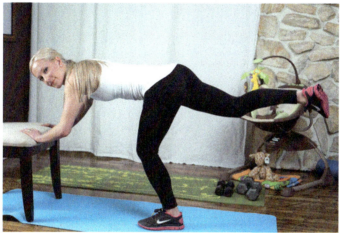

You come first photography

Exercise 13: Chair-assisted Glute Kick

Targets: glutes, legs, abdomen

You will need: a chair

10 repetitions (each leg)/3 Sets

Begin by facing the chair and placing both hands on the front of the seat and your left leg planted firmly on the floor. Keep your right leg off the ground and slightly bent toward your stomach. This is your starting position. While keeping your abdomen tight, extend the right leg all the way out behind you, squeezing the glutes. (Almost like you are trying to kick a door open.) Slowly bring back your right leg to starting position. Repeat.

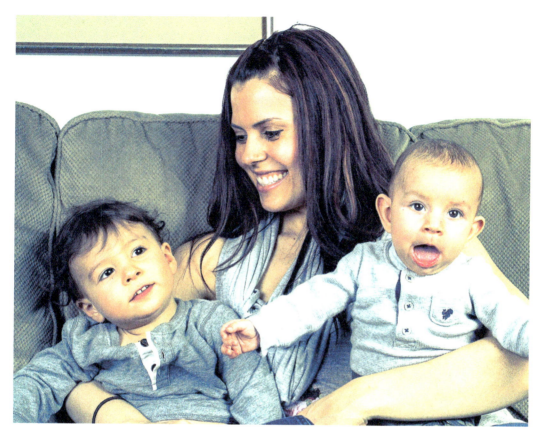

you come first photography

"Dedicated to my greatest inspiration, my Sons, Hunter and Mason"

Image Credits

1. AAdrianne Oyewole, UFIIT (www.ufiit.com)

2. Jeremy Martel, JM photography (www.JMportraits.ca)

3. Maggie Manchester, Pop Photography (popphotography@shaw.ca)

4. Shantel Hanson

5. Kimberly Denness-Thomas, Sweetgrass Images
https://www.facebook.com/sweetgrassfoto?fref=ts

6. Christian Benton, You Come First Photography (https://www.facebook.com/youcomefirstphotography)